IT'S NOT AS EASY AS I THOUGHT!

REVELATIONS ABOUT WORKING AND WELLNESS FROM A REAL WANDERER

Kristine Hudson

© 2020 Revelations About Working and Wellness from a Real Wanderer

All rights reserved. No part of the book may be reproduced in any shape or form without permission from the publisher.

This guide is written from a combination of experience and high-level research. Even though we have done our best to ensure this book is accurate and up to date, there are no guarantees to the accuracy or completeness of the contents herein.

This cover has been designed using resources from unsplash.com
ISBN: 978-1-953714-19-0

Reviews

Reviews and feedback help improve this book and the author. If you enjoy this book, we would greatly appreciate it if you could take a few moments to share your opinion and post a review on Amazon.

Contents

THINGS EVERY VAN LIFER NEEDS TO KNOW

Section 1: Making the Big Decision   11

    Chapter 1: Why Do I Want to Live in a Van?   12

    Chapter 2: The Reality of Van Living - Doing Your Homework   17

    Chapter 3: The Human Element of Van Life- Health and Wealth   22

        Advice from The Road- Part 1   26

Section 2: Finding Your New Home   31

    Chapter 1: Considerations for Choosing the Right Vehicle   31

    Chapter 2: So Many Choices!   37

    Chapter 3: Ready-to-Roll, or Ready-to-Rehab?   44

    Chapter 4: Budget Considerations for Creating Your Van   50

    Chapter 5: The Search Process   56

        Advice from the Road- Part 2   60

Section 3: Creating and Maintaining a Budget While on the Road   63

    Advice from the Road: Part 3   63

    Chapter 1: Determining Your Budget   65

        Advice from the Road: Part 4   69

    Chapter 2: Sticking to It   71

Chapter 3: Earning Income While on the Move	73
Advice from the Road: Part 5	74
Section 4: Preparing for Your Trip	77
Chapter 1: Your Utilities	77
Chapter 2: Sleeping Arrangements	78
Advice from the Road: Part 6	82
Chapter 3: Storage Solutions	82
Chapter 4: Emergency Kit	85
Chapter 5: Food	88
Section 5: Where Are You Going to Go?	95
Advice from the Road: Part 7	98
Section 6: Staying Happy on the Road	102
Chapter 1: Avoiding Boredom	102
Chapter 2: Homesickness/Loneliness	104
Advice from the Road: Part 8	105
Chapter 3: Housekeeping	106
In Conclusion	109
Section 7: Helpful Resources for Future Van Dwellers	113

WORK WHERE YOU WANT TO BE: HOW TO LEAVE THE OFFICE BEHIND

Section One: The Here and Now of Working on the Run — 121

    Introduction: Why Do I Need This Book? What Will I Learn? — 121

    Chapter One: My Own Journey to "Working on the Run" — 124

    Chapter Two: Where are you? An Excercise in learning more about yourself — 124

    Chapter Three: The Pros & Cons of Working Remotely — 135

    Chapter Four: What Will You Accomplish With This Change? — 138

Section Two: Details, Details, Details — 143

    Chapter One: Determining the Who, Where, When, and How of Working on the Run — 143

        Your Challenge: An Exercise in Reality — 144

    Chapter Two: Who, Where, and When- Just the Facts — 146

Section Three: What Will I Be? What Will I Do? — 155

    Chapter One: Same as It Ever Was — 156

    Chapter Two: Redefining the "Free" in "Freelancing" — 162

    Chapter Three: A Side-Hustle You Can Do All Day- or Not! — 166

Chapter Four: Here, There, and Everywhere	171
Chapter Five: Something for Everyone	173

Section Four: Setting the Stage — 175

Chapter One: Creating Your Work Space	175
Chapter Two: Understanding How to Work in a New Place	180
Chapter Three: Time to Work!	183

Section Four: Finding Your Stride and Making It Work — 189

Chapter One: The Social Aspect	189
Chapter Two: The Growth Aspect	193
Chapter Three: The Financial Aspect	196
Chapter Four: The Fear Aspect	198

Section Five: Wrapping It All Up — 205

Section 6: Resources for Former Office Workers — 211

Productivity Management Resources	211
Money Management Resources	212
Technical Resources	213
Network/Community Resources	216

HOW TO LIVE THE DREAM:

THINGS EVERY VAN LIFER NEEDS TO KNOW

Kristine Hudson

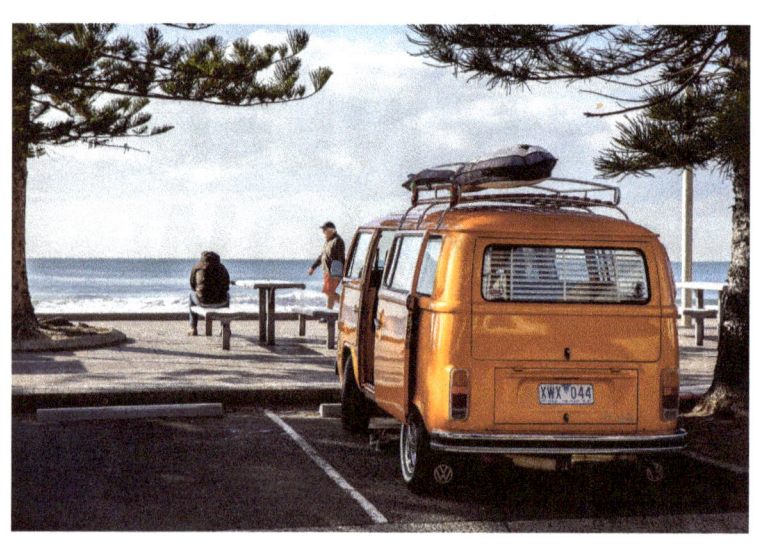

Section 1: Making the Big Decision

There's a certain romance to the idea of living on the road. Traveling wherever the wind blows. Leaving nothing except footprints. Taking nothing but pictures.

The media is awash with images of attractive, wind-swept people, staring out of their windows at an awe-inspiring vista. Mountains, oceans, and fields so far and wide, you can hardly see the horizon. All these images make van living look like an incredible option. Not only do you get to shed the boring, stale, workaday lifestyle, but you get to wake up wherever you want.

To many, van living is the ultimate goal. It is the dream that just won't go away. While there's tons of material in the media explaining how amazing van life is, there is little to help you prepare for the reality of life on the road.

We'll explore what it takes to hack a nomadic lifestyle in the 21st century, with road tips provided from actual American van dwellers. Throughout this book, you'll find "Advice from the Road," which contains tips, tricks, and details provided by folks who have personally practiced the van lifestyle.

We'll start with all the considerations you'll need to keep in mind before making the decision to follow your wanderlust. We'll also go through the process of choosing your new home, as well as things to consider when creating and utilizing space. Budgeting, as well as managing income and expenditures, is also a huge part of van life. We'll help you get packed and ready to hit the trails, with some tips and tricks for staying happy and learning to find your home on the road.

You might be surprised at how involved the process is, but bear in mind that this is always your adventure. You can ramp up or tame the journey to meet your preferred lifestyle. After all, this is *your* life's dream!

Chapter 1: Why Do I Want to Live in a Van?

Before you start the engine and bid farewell to your friends and family — before you even have an engine to start — you must get in touch with your dream. This may sound a bit New Age, but the reality is that you are about to commit to a very significant lifestyle change by living in a van. Whether you have a regular nine-to-five job that you're sick of, or have been a freewheeling freelancer for years, van living is nothing like what you have experienced to date.

You will not be able to come home. If you have a rough day, you won't be able to "just stay in and order a pizza." The routines that have come to rule your life will no longer exist.

If hearing that makes your heart beat a little faster, you're not alone. The primary reason people choose van life is because they are sick of having a home and a yard, or an apartment and neighbors. They're tired of commuting to work. They don't want to spend an entire weekend cleaning floors and dusting knick-knacks. They want to live.

If you identify with this, you're on the right track. But here's one important question to ask yourself: By living on the road, what do you hope to achieve? What deep, burning need in your life will van living satisfy, and are you prepared to make a significant number of sacrifices to find that lifestyle?

Let us point out before you start feeling less certain about van living: there are different types of van living experiences.

First, there's the type of Van Lifers who maintain their home and daily lifestyle but use their van as a mobile escape. In previous decades, truly adventurous families had vacation properties, such as beach condos or lakeside cabins. The modern twist on this is to make the holiday home a van, so adventure may take place anywhere you can imagine to drive.

Then there are the semi-permanent nomads. These folks may have a PO Box in a permanent location. They may live full time in the van, but they stay tied to a particular area, whether that be an RV park, long-term campground, or the general vicinity. They may take off for an adventure now and again, but they migrate only around a certain radius.

Lastly, there are the true devotees. These folks plan to see as much as possible and do as much as they can before their time on this planet expires. They hope to never see the same sunset or sunrise — though if they do, they maintain it's purely because they wanted to see that view one more time. These folks don't plan to land on terra firma any time soon and are fully prepared to have all their needs fulfilled by life on the road.

You may fit firmly within one of these categories. You might find yourself somewhere in shades in between. Remember, there is no "wrong way" to organize your dreams. The goal of van life is to fulfill a need you have deep in your soul, and if your soul decides it wants to come home and do a load of laundry, that does not mean you're not accomplishing your dream.

When it comes to van living, there are a few aspects of the lifestyle that tend to be magnets to most people considering the option. Let's explore those in more detail.

The Chance to Live Off-Grid
While "keeping up with the Joneses'" has been part of the American Dream for over a century, there are many who are no longer impressed with this ideal. A larger house might be a great fantasy, but that involves a heftier house payment — which means working more hours. And a bigger house means more "stuff," like furniture and decorations. Owning more means increased upkeep, higher utility bills, taking care of a bigger lawn, etc. For some folks, this sounds less like the American Dream and more like a terrifying nightmare.

A van does not have a mortgage, though you might find yourself making payments on your roaming home — we'll discuss that more later. A van doesn't have utility bills. A van doesn't have an attic to maintain or a basement that floods when it rains. A van doesn't have noisy neighbors. You will do no yard work.

But that doesn't mean it's completely carefree. A van is a mechanical invention, and it can break down. Windows can crack. Tires can blow. You'll need to find new ways of creating power. You will not have running water unless you create that option. If anything breaks, you will have to take care of it, and immediately. While van living does mean you'll be living off the grid, it does not mean you'll live without responsibility.

The Ability to Be Self-Sustaining
Urban and suburban lifestyles require constant connection. You have neighbors. You have coworkers. You have friends. Your social obligations require you to continually connect with these individuals in order to sustain your network and relationships. How much time do you have to yourself?

Traveling the country solo, with just the wind as your copilot may seem like the best way to completely disconnect and shed all these social responsibilities. You have the chance to be alone with your own mind and learn who you are. You can discover how your mind and soul work, and uncover the mystery of who you want to become before your time on this planet draws to a close.

When you work 40-80 hours a week, 52 weeks of the year, you lose the connection with yourself and become the routine that maintains your lifestyle. Being on the road will tear you away from what you've known as life, and guide you to understanding who you really are.

And that means completely upending that routine. What will you do on Saturday mornings, if not going to meet friends for brunch, followed by cleaning the bathroom? When Monday morning arrives, how will you greet the day if you don't have to shower and get ready for work before the sun rises?

For many of us, our lifestyle is determined by what we need to do to keep doing the same thing. When you live on the road, you no longer have to sustain these patterns. While you certainly can continue to work in an office if that's your preference, you won't feel the pressure to work 12-hour days to pay the bills. It certainly won't take you multiple hours to clean the bathroom. Every aspect of your life will be simplified to the most basic needs, rather than creating a level of comfort.

Will you be able to live without guidelines, restrictions, or limitations of someone else? Will you choose instead to learn how to self-sustain, the way humans were intended to live?

The Freedom to Roam
When you no longer live under the demands of someone else's schedule, you have the ability to create your own agenda. This means you can go anywhere you want. You can see what you want to see. Do what you want to do. You don't have to be in the boardroom for a meeting at 3 pm every day. You don't have to take a day off work to wait for the repair technician because the cable isn't working. You have the freedom to dictate your own schedule, and your home has four rubber wheels that are designed to take you anywhere.

This may sound absolutely ideal for many, but it can also cause a bit of anxiety for others. Choice paralysis is real, and some people might have a hard time deciding what to do next. After all, hunting and gathering is no longer a truly viable option in the United States, so following the herds and water sources is not a requirement for survival.

The freedom to roam also means you have to decide where you're going to go. You may be the type of person who has to know where you're going to be on any given day, and that's a hard habit to break. When it is midnight and you're driving through a severe thunderstorm, you might regret not having found a place to park and turn in for the night. After all, though you may shed the responsibilities of suburban life, you'll never get past biological needs!

Even at its most liberating, van life still demands a certain amount of planning and research. While you'll have the ability to go anywhere you want, you still have to acknowledge the practicalities, legalities, and realities that await you.

See the World on Your Own Time
Now that you are no longer living under someone else's agenda, you have to create your own. This doesn't have to be a hard-set "to-do" list of daily chores, but instead, a list of goals and accomplishments you'd like to have under your belt in time.

Before you hit the road, create a list of places you'd like to see, or things you'd like to do. Want to summit El Capitan? Fantastic. Have a burning desire to see the sun rise on the southernmost point of the country? Excellent. Consider themes and key points of interest that really get your blood pumping. Now that you have this freedom, it's time to make the most of it.

Once you are on the road, you truly have the ability to see the world. If you choose to make van living a full-time lifestyle, then this is not a vacation. You do not have to be back in the office in three days' time. You don't need to hire someone to water the plants. If you are going to be a part-time road warrior, however, then you will need to adjust accordingly, which makes having an agenda even more important. After all, the reason you've chosen to live in a van, instead of a tiny house or exotic cave, is because you embrace mobility.

Consider the Alternative
Now that you've really defined why you feel compelled to live in a van, consider the option of not living in a van.

That's right — the time has come to ask yourself why this is so important. One way to make your desires truly transparent is to look at the situation from the flip side.

What if you don't pursue this? What if you just stay home, continue working your job, making sure your knick-knacks don't get dusty? Maybe you go camping every weekend to scratch that wanderlust itch, but you don't go all the way into van living. Would this be something that you would regret?

Living in a van is demanding. Physically, you'll find you have to spend a significant amount of time driving. Your gym routine is likely a thing of the past, too, and you'll have to find ways to feed yourself that don't involve a full-sized kitchen. Emotionally, you will be alone with your thoughts, all day, every day. Are you prepared to keep yourself entertained? Are you comfortable addressing all of the thoughts, hopes, dreams, and emotions that have been ignored while you go with the urban flow? Mentally, you're going to have to prepare for a new set of dangers and challenges. While remaining open to rewards that would never be possible when living in a two bedroom walk-up.

Successful van life is more than just knowing how to set up your bathroom and innovative storage. It is far more than dangling tan legs out the window or watching the sun rise and set in new, amazing places. This is an opportunity to shed not only your electric bill, but every expectation that has ever been made of you and your abilities. You will need to learn a new set of survival skills, and the things that made you feel "comfortable" in a home-dwelling lifestyle will no longer be the same.

In many ways, van living is an entirely new life, and this is a journey that will require dedication and preparation in order to serve you well. You will learn much along the way; in fact, many would argue that you'll learn far more about life when living on the road. However, you have to be prepared to execute those skills and to be ready for a new set of challenges.

Chapter 2: The Reality of Van Living - Doing Your Homework

Before making the decision to commit to van life, it is important that you understand all the challenges and potential hazards that come with the lifestyle. While you have a new and exciting level of freedom, you are going to encounter a new level of responsibility. Not only do you have complete control over where you roam, but you are required to solve every problem that might arise.

This is not to say these problems are too hard to solve. In fact, being prepared before you hit the road will help turn these problems into a variety of inconveniences, rather than taking all the zest out of van living. You will find that one of the key elements to a successful van lifestyle is planning and preparation, which can begin as soon as you start day-dreaming about the possibilities.

Let's look at some of the key areas in which you'll need to practice good planning and preparation. This includes: knowing how to keep up with van maintenance, being aware of your equipment, keeping it in good working order, and finding places to park and catch up on rest.

Van Maintenance

Taking care of yourself will be critical on the road, but taking care of your van will be equally important. Therefore, you will need to learn some basic van maintenance.

There are many aspects of vehicle repair and preservation that are relatively simple and can be conducted on nearly any flat service. Being able to check, monitor, and replenish your fluids is a great place to start. Oil, coolant, transmission fluid, brake fluid, and power steering fluid are all things that will need constant observation when you live on the road. They need very little automotive skill to learn where to find the input point, what type to buy, and when to top off your supply.

You may want to invest a little more effort into your overall maintenance skills in order to preserve your overall autonomy. There are two basic facts that apply to any van living situation:
1. A vehicle in motion will require more maintenance, more frequently.
2. Vans require specialized mechanics in many cases. Some vans have a different type of mechanical engineering, and others are

too heavy for a regular repair shop's lift system. In either case, you will not be able to simply roll your van up to any mechanic's shop for basic maintenance.

These two reasons make a compelling case for learning how to do your own basic vehicle care, such as changing oil and oil filters, as well as air filters and fuel filters. While finding a mechanic who can work on your van might be tricky, finding an auto parts store that carries the items you need is far less challenging.

Knowing your vehicle inside and out isn't entirely necessary, especially if you have a particular mechanical ineptitude; however, you will want to become familiar enough with your van to diagnose certain issues. You may want to consider a few automotive classes or online courses. You can also enhance your knowledge or learning process by checking out online videos, which you can bookmark for future reference.

Once you have learned the basic mechanical anatomy and processes of your vehicle, you will want to keep several references in your vehicle at all times. The first is the owner's manual. It can be somewhat tricky to track down owner's manuals, especially if you are purchasing an older vehicle or one that has already gone through several rounds of remodels or rehabs. However, you should be able to find supplemental information online that can provide key information on motors, as well as years, makes, and models of a variety of vehicles.

In addition to the owner's manual, you will want a repair handbook specific to your vehicle type. Understanding the basics in your vehicle could save you hundreds of dollars and days of possible lost time, simply by being able to identify where the problem is.

Lastly, you will need to keep immaculate maintenance records of your own. Not only will this help you track when you need regular preventive care, like oil changes and tire rotations, but can help you record any patterns or trouble areas, such as brakes wearing down too quickly or hoses needing replacing more frequently than you imagined.

As you learn about your vehicle, pay attention to what tools you'll need to fix common repair techniques. Often these tools will be useful for a variety of maintenance in and around the van and will become part of your onboard kit.

Your Key Equipment

While we'll discuss the type of equipment you'll need in your van further in Section 2 and 3, it is important to note that you will also be responsible for the care and maintenance of the equipment within your van.

This can include everything from your cooking surface to your water and power systems, to your most low-tech equipment, such as a cooler or tent.

When living in a van, you do not have the luxury of packing loads of supplies. Instead, you have limited space and thus need to pack only necessary gear, and tools essential for the repair of that gear. For example, instead of packing a main tent and a spare, a better use of space is to pack a tent and a tent repair kit.

You may also be limited as to what you can easily replace. Buying new screens for your windows may seem tempting, but your budget will dictate whether you can do this. Instead, consider learning how to repair the equipment that you will have onboard.

This will likely mean investing in tools and common repair elements, such as tarps, duct tape, twine, and more. As you learn how each piece of equipment in your van works, learn how it can fail to function and what you'll need to have onboard to keep it in good working order. Again, this will save you hundreds of dollars and tons of frustration.

Locations for Landing

At some point in your day, you will need to rest. Your van will also likely thank you for the break. Therefore, you will need to know where, when, and how long you can park your van in a variety of locations. After all, getting a ticket or threatened with towing will put a real damper on your experience... and budget.

Unfortunately, "free parking" is more a thing of the past in inhabited areas. Loiterers and an influx of illegal activity have really put a damper on being able to park and sleep for the night. However, there are some locations in which you'll be able to catch at least a few hours of shut-eye.

Some retail locations — especially stores that supply outdoor activities — still permit adventurers of all kinds a few hours to rest in their parking lots. Before you make assumptions, however, be sure to check with store management to understand the parameters of their offerings. Also, you'll always want to obey posted signage. Sometimes the business does not own the parking lot, so separate rules will apply to those traveling through.

Truck stops and rest areas are other popular spots for a quick rest. Again, there may be time limits on your stay. Always obey posted signs and local ordinances. These will generally be posted in a common area of the rest stop.

Another fantastic resource for free parking is National Land. This refers to land within National Forests or territory that is not otherwise owned or maintained by a private owner. The majority of this land lies west of the Mississippi River, and can be a fantastic opportunity for van people. While these are not paved or maintained sites, and they will not feature luxuries such as even the most remote vault toilet, you can find flat, remote places where you can legally park for free. Once again, there may be limits on how long you can stay in these spots.

Finding spots to park may seem like a game of roulette, but there are actually many resources available to help you hunt down options. (These have been included in the **Resource Guide** at the end of the book.) Van people are, above all, sympathetic to each others' quests and willing to help out whenever possible. Therefore, a wealth of information can be found online or even by talking to others on the road.

Van living does require knowledge and skills, beyond that which you may have at the outset of planning your new lifestyle. However, keep in mind that any lifestyle has a learning curve. When you moved into your house, for example, you probably had to learn where all the light switches were, or how to get the hot water to work. Van living is a very similar experience — you need to learn a new skill set. But once learned, it will help you immeasurably and become part of your daily rituals.

Chapter 3: The Human Element of Van Life- Health and Wealth

Besides requiring a certain amount of mechanical know-how, there are quite a few existential challenges you will encounter on the road, which require mental preparation before you embark on your new mobile lifestyle.

One thing to keep in mind is that you are by and large in control of your overall experience. Everything you have, you make happen. You will no longer have the opportunity to walk over to the neighbor's house to borrow a cup of sugar. You will need to be prepared for everything the road throws at you.

At the same time, do not be bogged down by responsibility. While van living is a totally different type of lifestyle, in time, it will become second nature. Just as you had to figure out life in your first apartment or how to adapt to your first job; you will learn to live in a van. However, be gentle with yourself and allow yourself time to get comfortable with the notion. In the early days, you may question your decision or find yourself unsure of what to do next. This is normal. We all experience growing pains and a learning curve whenever we make huge changes in our lives.

To begin, you can prepare for your new lifestyle before you even purchase your van. Not only can you learn maintenance procedures and parking regulations, but you can prepare yourself for the challenges you'll face as a human as well.

Your Health

In addition to taking care of your van and equipment, you will need to take care of yourself while you are on the road. Not only will your body need to be fed when it is hungry, have access to adequate clean water, and rest when necessary, but you will need regular maintenance as well. Staying in perfect health becomes more complicated when you are on the road. You will be exposed to a new world of germs, and you won't be able to visit your regular doctor if you start feeling under the weather.

There are many things you can do, to ensure your health is always a priority:

1. Pack a first aid kit, including care for multiple types of wounds and injuries. This includes bandages, wraps, antiseptic cream, absorbent pads, athletic wrap and tape, as well as instant ice packs and heat packs.
2. Pack a wellness kit, too. This can include cold medicine, over-the-counter products for pain and fever, topical cream for sprains and strains, throat lozenges, sleep aids, and products for heartburn or upset stomachs.
3. Consider a daily vitamin. Even with a refrigeration system, you won't be able to have full, immediate access to all the fresh fruit and vegetables you had at home, so make sure your body and immune system are fully prepared.
4. If you are on any daily prescriptions, talk to your prescribing physician before you hit the road. You may wish to transfer your prescriptions to a national pharmacy chain and purchase prescriptions in 90-day supplies whenever possible. Often, this will require your doctor's approval. Also share with your doctor where you will be traveling, as some states do not permit non-residents to pick up certain prescriptions. You do not want

to suffer the side effects of missed essential medication while on the road, as that can quickly become serious. Planning ahead with your doctor will ensure you are ahead of the game.
5. Illness will happen. Before you hit the road, consider what your backup plan will be in case you are too sick to drive for several days. Hotels and long-term parking facilities can be expensive but may prove necessary when you are sick. The alternative of driving while you are unable has far greater consequences.
6. Consider your insurance situation, as well. What will happen if you need to go to the hospital, emergency room, or urgent care? In the United States, private insurance is often a requirement to offset very high expenses. What is your plan for carrying insurance during your travels?

Mental Wellness

In addition to your physical well-being, consider your mental health, as well. Being on the road is not always fun! The road will bring more rewards than regrets, but there will be days when you are stationary because of maintenance, sickness, or complacency. There will be days when you "just don't wanna." If you have a "go, go, go" type of plan, there may come a time when you want to "rest, rest, rest." You will need to listen to your mind and body when these days happen because your health is always going to be a huge factor in your overall success on the road.

What will you do when the weather is bad? You might have a day of hiking washed out by unexpected thunderstorms. You may plan to do some maintenance but find yourself unable to do so on a foggy day. Things will not always go as planned, and sometimes the impeding factor is the weather itself. You will likely not want to spend the day confined in your van, which means you'll need to learn how to play along with Mother Nature. Not only will you need a solid weather app, but weather gear, as well. There are certain points in the United States where snow exists year-round. There are also locations where the temperatures can reach over 100 degrees.

Besides being prepared with equipment, make sure you're mentally ready for bad weather, too. If it's going to rain, perhaps you find a local, free museum. If the temperatures are going to be incredibly high, sleep during the day and drive at night to avoid overheating yourself and your van.

Additionally, boredom is real. Finding structure will help you prevent this, but it's going to happen. You might have a daily ritual, but even that will become tedious at times. Even when you find yourself driving to your next adventure, you might find yourself sick of driving and tired of listening to the same old music. This is natural. Don't take boredom as a sign of failure. Instead, pull over and find a new station, podcast, or audiobook. Perhaps you can take some time to catch up on your housekeeping and organization. Maybe you pause and write down how you're feeling. Do a search online for somewhere nearby to take a stroll and clear your thoughts.

When you feel this way at home, what do you do? Most likely, you throw on some television, or call your friends, or find something around the house to occupy your time. You can still do these things on the road, too! It's entirely ok to feel burnt out on driving all the time. Allow yourself downtime, and when you find yourself feeling bored of that, seek out new ways to occupy your time. Consider picking up games and activity books or coloring books. What about journaling? If you're a creator, you can still paint, knit, and craft on the road, or dabble in whatever your preferred media is. Anything you can do to occupy your time can be done in a van, as long as you're willing to change the scale. For example, you won't be able to throw an entire pottery wheel and kiln on your van, but you can grab some modeling clay and play with making tiny creations that will exercise your talent and creativity.

Your Wealth

Despite not having fixed bills, van living can be expensive. Prepare for this now. Before you start budgeting — which we'll discuss in another section — you need to know what types of expenses you can encounter. This includes everything from mechanical breakdowns and flat tires, to daily expenses, like gasoline, food, water, and generator operation. Parking permits cost money, and showering on the road can cost money too (if you don't have a water supply onboard). Every cup of coffee you purchase at a gas station dips into your budget.

If you plan to make van living your full-time lifestyle, what will you do for income? Many employers offer the opportunity to work remotely, which can be a huge benefit, depending on your profession. This also means you'll likely need to be sure you have a functioning laptop and a reliable Wi-Fi signal. While more and more public locations offer free Wi-Fi, consider if you'll really want to spend every day in a new coffee shop or home improvement store parking lot borrowing signal in order to send in a big report. Instead, you may wish to invest in a web connection amplifier or booster, so that you can run your office right from your van.

You may instead decide to do freelance work on the road. You'll be surrounded by infinite muses, so if you are able to do so, make it happen! You can also run a blog or livestream your journey. Again, this will require a Wi-Fi signal and likely a handful of equipment, so be sure you have a solid plan in place before you set up your van. Having an adequate workspace in your van will definitely increase your professional success.

Van living is incredibly rewarding; however, it does include a bit of adaptation, especially if you've lived a relatively sedentary, domestic life. You may feel like a proverbial fish out of water for some time, but this does not mean you're "doing it wrong." In fact, it means you're finally spreading your wings and finding your groove.

Advice from The Road- Part 1

I hate to be the bearer of bad news, but everything is going to go wrong. Not necessarily all at once, but don't rule that out!

When we hit the road, we started slowly. We started with a two week trip around the vicinity of our home. We wanted to make sure that, no matter what happened, we would be within a reasonable distance of our actual home, so we could "come back" if everything proved to be too much. That included too expensive, too scary, too unpredictable… if at any point we got overwhelmed, we could dart back home and say we had a very nice, short vacation.

Everything went according to plan. We saw the sights, we took the back roads, we gathered loads of amazing photographs and memories. Then, just nine hours away from home, everything went sideways. Huge mechanical breakdown — one of those situations where one thing breaks, and then all the bits and pieces around it start breaking. It was beyond anything we could take care of ourselves because so many things were just falling apart.

Worse yet — we were supposed to be in a wedding at home in just two days!

We had the choice of trying to find someone who could help fix it, or just abandon our van, find a rental car, and figure out how to get the van back later. It took all day, but we were able to find — and get the van to — a mechanic. Even then, it wasn't fixable without ordering parts that would take several days to arrive.

Thankfully, the mechanic was sympathetic to van life. He'd done it himself. Since he couldn't fix it, he came up with a suitable workaround that would get us home. He also recommended that, once we started driving, we not stop except for fuel.

We thought we were home free but still fell prey to the mayhem that can be road life. Even when you think things are going well, it just takes one situation to remind you that "fine" is a temporary state of mind.

Still, there's nothing I'd give up about life on the road. Bad things happen in an apartment. Your car can break down on the way to the office. Your milk will go bad, and your dog will barf in your shoes.

A Van Lifer is someone who can adapt, overcome, and think of creative situations to nearly every problem. Furthermore, they accept that sometimes the solution is "ask an expert." Van Life is a community effort, even if that community is constantly moving in different directions!

Did we get back on the road? Absolutely! We had to spend a bit more time at home than we planned, getting the parts we needed, but that gave us time to learn more about the situation and research solutions for when (not if) it happened again.

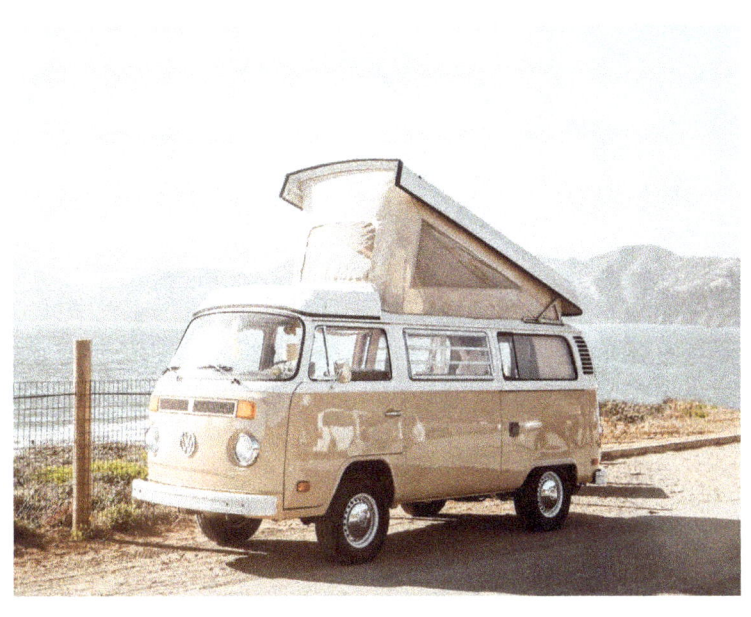

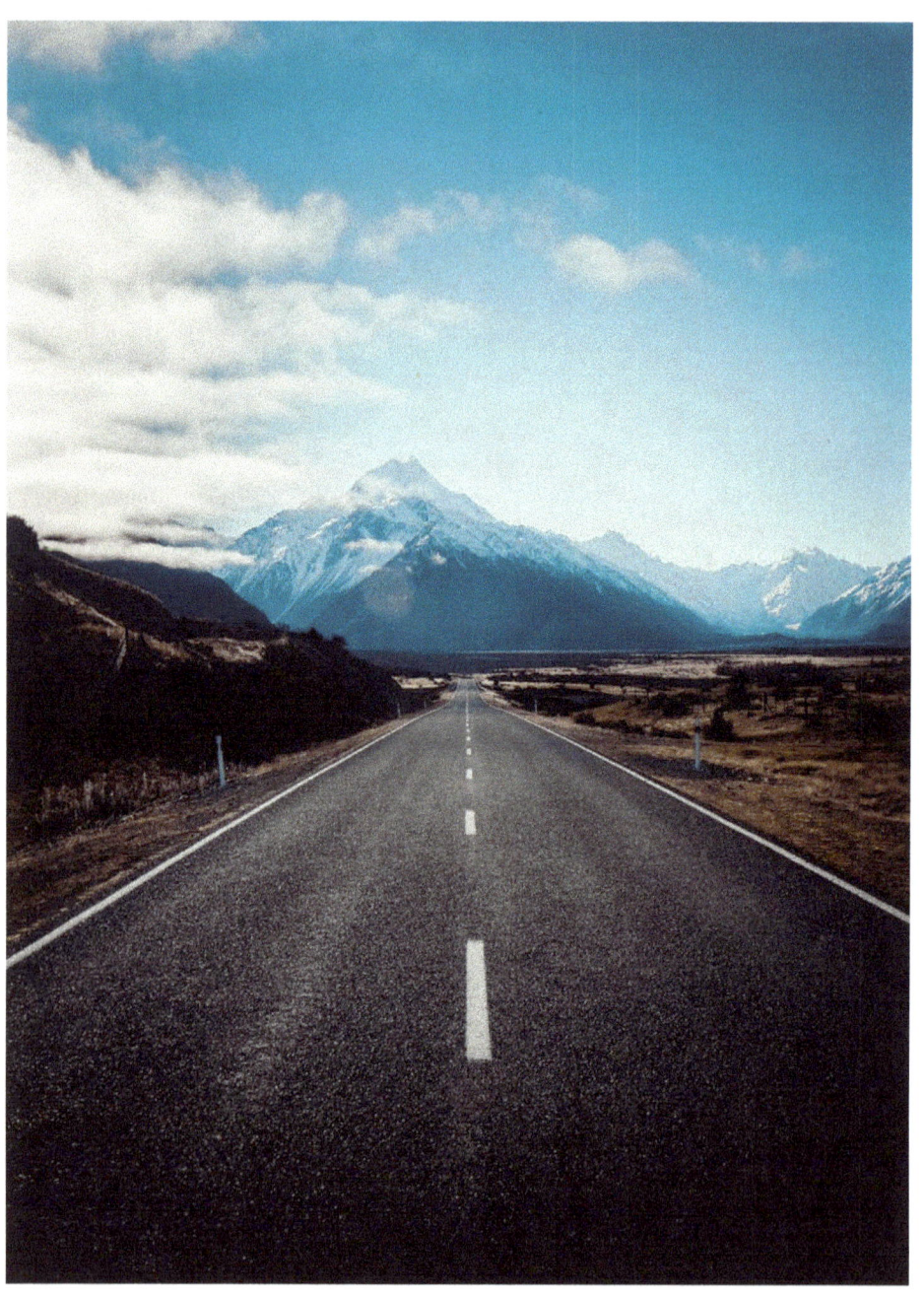

Section 2: Finding Your New Home

Being aware of what it takes to successfully live on the road is all well and good, but once you have your mind made up, it's time to find the chariot that will carry you through all of life's adventures.

Again, you might take to the internet to find pictures of vans with white-washed walls, gleaming hardwood floors, tile backsplashes, and even wood-burning stoves. Looks awfully cozy, doesn't it?

While you can make these beautiful images part of your reality, the truth is that it will take a lot of work to get there.

In this section, we'll look at the different things you need to keep in mind when choosing your new vehicle, as well as how to proceed with converting your van into your dream home.

Chapter 1: Considerations for Choosing the Right Vehicle

If you look at any Van Life-themed social media account, you'll find that the term "van" is somewhat open to interpretation. You'll see a fair share of classic vans, such as Volkswagen Vanagons, Westphalia, and Transporters. You'll also see conversion vans, cargo vans, and European camper vans. But the lifestyle also extends to "skoolies," or converted school buses. This, in turn, has inspired folks to convert buses of all kinds. Inventive folks have also taken to converting campers from part-time vacation homes to full-time homes on wheels.

So, when you start searching for your new home, you might be completely stalled at how many options are available. In a nutshell, your decision will be driven by a lot of personal factors. Let's examine these further.

Determining Vehicle Size

There's a considerable amount of difference in size between a skoolie and a VW Transporter, just as there's a huge difference between a three-bedroom house and a studio apartment.

One of the first things you'll need to consider is how much space you need. There are a lot of elements that can go into this part of your accommodations.

1. The number of passengers — and their species!
2. The length of the trip
3. The amenities, such as a bathroom, food preparation area, etc
4. Personal preference

The number of passengers will, of course, dictate how many seats and how many sleeping areas you will need in your van. If you'll have children with you, you might feel most comfortable if they're able to be safely belted into fixed seats while the vehicle is moving. While nearly every veteran van lifer has an amusing story of using a cooler as a seat, it's frowned upon by the law and definitely not safe!

If you're bringing your Adventure Pup or a Feline Mascot (neither of which is unheard of!), you'll have to plan to accommodate their needs, as well. For dogs, you'll want to make sure you have room for them to rest while you drive, move around as they wish when they're not on an adventure with you, and a spot for them to sleep. This can mean making room for a dog bed or making room in your bed for a dog. Cats typically need around 16-18 square feet of space to feel comfortable. They'll also need a litter pan that won't slosh all over the floor of the van unless otherwise toilet trained. Many people do share their van life with a furry friend, so it can be done, with careful planning!

The second part of determining space from the number of passengers is based on comfort level. If you are currently sharing a three-bedroom house with two children and a dog, You're accustomed to a certain amount of space in which to maneuver. Even in the largest bus, you will still run into each other, and you will find privacy a very rare element, indeed. However, if you're currently sharing a studio with your partner, then you're already well-prepared for the challenges that come with cohabitating in a tiny space.

The length of the trip will also dictate the size of vehicle you need, if largely from the standpoint of accommodating four seasons worth of equipment and clothing. If you plan on making your van your permanent home, then you'll need to consider how you'll plan for the seasonal changes. Perhaps you take the opportunity to "chase the weather" and always park somewhere where the weather is dry and warm. Perhaps you choose a vehicle with additional storage for rain gear, snow gear, heavier blankets or sleeping bags, and fans for hot weather.

If you have the opportunity to stop and regroup periodically through your trip, you won't need to stash as much stuff. If you have a small storage unit (or a friend or relative who's willing to let you borrow some space), you can swing by as the situation calls for to change out your equipment, clothing, and more. Granted, this means you'll have to plan ahead to drive to that specific location in time, but it can save you hundreds of pounds and several square feet of extra "stuff" you don't need to carry with you everywhere.

The next consideration is how you will use the room within your vehicle. If you plan to have a bathroom area, you're likely going to want a camper- or bus-type set up. If you instead plan to pack a portable toilet and bucket-style shower, you can really make any type of vehicle work. We'll discuss this in more detail shortly, but at this stage, you'll want to consider if you want to have a full water closet with plumbing or if you can deal with an alternative plan.

The same is true for food preparation areas. The most rugged vans might have a cooler and a propane burner. The most luxurious have full oven ranges, small refrigerators, kitchen sinks, and cabinets. In between are an almost infinite variety of choices. We'll discuss kitchen needs and practical applications in a later section too, but at this stage, consider how much room you feel will be necessary for the kind of food prep you plan. If you're going to install plumbing, gas, or electricity for this, it's best to think of it now.

Lastly, your own personal preferences are something you truly need to consider. On paper, a solo voyager needs only a driver's seat and a bed, with room for storage. In reality, you might find yourself feeling very claustrophobic. The opposite can be true, too. You might find yourself overwhelmed by the size of your space and the maintenance required to keep it clean and functional.

One practical test that is recommended by all sorts of van life experts is the "try it at home" test. Before purchasing a van, bus, or camper of any kind, look up the approximate dimensions of space within the vehicle. Next, find a space in your home, garage, yard, basement, etc., and tape off those exact dimensions. Some experts recommend hanging sheets or shower curtains to give the illusion of the van walls, but you may be able to get a feel for what you'll be working with without going that far.

Without anything in it, how does this space feel? Now start adding objects to the area, either figuratively by marking off the space with tape or chalk, or literally. How big is the sleeping area? If you take that portion away, how well can you maneuver in the remaining space? There will be a learning curve when you actually start living in a van, but if you feel uncomfortable with the space before it's even "real," then you'll definitely want to consider a different option.

Another thing to keep in mind is the height of the van. If you're going with a regular-style van that does not have a pop-top, you may not be able to stand fully upright in the back. For those who are planning to use the van only as a place to sleep and store things, this might be perfectly acceptable. For others, this might be extremely limiting. Again, this comes down to personal preference, but it is definitely something you'll want to consider before you invest in your new home on wheels.

Vehicle Specifications
Beyond the considerations of space, there is the fact that you will have to drive this vehicle from time to time!

Of course, size is a consideration when operating a vehicle, as well. You should feel comfortable driving your van, camper, or bus in a variety of conditions, including on regular city streets, on the highway, on unmaintained or unpaved roads, and also be able to park and reverse.

While your particular trip might not include all of these elements, there will be times when something unforeseen occurs, and you'll need to make do. For example, there are parts of the country where the detour for a temporarily closed well-traveled road is a dirt path. Additionally, you might find it necessary to hit the freeway to get to the next closest gas station, even if you've carefully planned to avoid cities as much as possible. Therefore, it's important to be able to safely guide your vehicle wherever you happen to roam.

If you plan to frequently encounter those unmaintained and unpaved roads, you'll also want to pay close attention to your drivetrain. A drivetrain contains the parts (components) of a vehicle that deliver power to certain wheels.

Let's look at the differences:

- Two-wheel drive (2WD). If your van is referred to as "rear-wheel drive" or "front-wheel drive," it's a 2WD model.
    - Rear-wheel drive delivers the power to the back wheels, and thus the vehicle is "pushed" forward from behind, so the front wheels can handle steering. Many sports cars are RWD, resulting in a balanced, powerful drive. On the flip side, RWD vehicles perform poorly in wet or freezing conditions.
    - Front-wheel drive delivers power to the front wheels, where the engine weight provides balance that improves overall traction. These vehicles typically have a more respectable fuel economy, as well, which can be important to your budget.

- Four-wheel drive (4WD). This option allows drivers to select between RWD and 4WD, depending on the terrain. 4WD delivers power to all four wheels simultaneously, which is fantastic when taking on tough terrain but terrible for your fuel economy. This is why engineers offer the ability to turn off 4WD when the conditions don't require it.
- All-wheel drive (AWD). This option is becoming more and more popular with larger vehicles. AWD requires a front, rear, and central differential, which means all four wheels have power when they need it. A lot of modern (post-2015) heavy-duty vehicles offer this type of drivetrain as an option. Automatic AWD operates in 2WD until the computer sensors determine extra power is needed in a specific location. It is unlikely that you will find this feature on a bus or older van, however.

The rest of the vehicle options you'll need to choose between are far more intuitive. Do you want an engine that runs on regular gasoline or diesel? Check the specifications for any vehicle you're interested in to determine what kind of fuel it needs, as well as the overall fuel economy.

What about transmission? Can you drive a standard, or will an automatic transmission be the best option for you and any others who will be along for the trip? While fans of each option can debate the merits and downfalls of each for eternity, the reality, in this case, is that you'll need to be able to choose a van you can regularly drive without issue.

Insurance

We won't go into too much detail on this topic because requirements and options vary from state to state and country to country. Still, insurance is a very important part of the equation. Not only will you need to have insurance on your vehicle if you plan to drive anywhere, but you'll want to make sure your contents are covered, as well.

Before you purchase any van, bus, or camper, speak with your insurance representative. You'll want to make sure you're covered not only as a driver but also for any accidents that might befall your new home. There are plenty of situations that might render your vehicle undrivable or your quarters unliveable. You need to make sure you're protected not just on the road but for your lifestyle, as well.

When you speak to your insurance representative, make sure you bring up all of these concerns and receive a quote. You will need to decide if you prefer to budget for a higher level of insurance coverage or put away enough savings as a cushion for any mishaps that occur. While it may seem early to think about this, it's crucial that you are able to afford the insurance on any vehicle you might take out on the road. Otherwise, it's simply not the vehicle for you!

Chapter 2: So Many Choices!

If you were to type the word "van" into Google, you'd probably get far, far more information than you could rationally digest in one sitting. Therefore, we'll quickly run through the different types of vehicles you might consider, as well as some factors that might go into your decision to purchase — or stay far away from — that type.

There are plenty of nuances and adaptations to each and every individual van, so it would be impossible to review every single brand that has ever been used for van life. Instead, we'll look at the overall classes of van, and remember — these are just basic guidelines. As they say on the road, "Your Mileage May Vary!"

Classic Vans

These are your Vanagons, your Westphalia, Transporters, and all of the Instagram-ready VW campers that fit the expected stereotype. This class can also include any pre-1990 vans from any manufacturer.

Speaking from an aesthetic point of view, these vehicles are often very photogenic and will get tons of attention on the road. They've got that "old school" appeal that dredges up pleasant, nostalgic memories in nearly anyone who traveled extensively in childhood.

There is, in fact, a huge community of Classic Van Lifers, so you'll be able to connect with plenty of folks who have extensively driven, maintained, rehabbed, worked on, lived in, or are in any possible way familiar with these vans. This is great news for anyone new to van life because you'll have plenty of resources and support through each step of the process.

In fact, when shopping for a Classic Van, you'll find that a large portion of those for sale will be more or less road-ready, due to the fact that many people have purchased and rehabbed these vehicles, then moved on to a bigger and better project following the success of their maiden voyage.

Also, thanks to the recent resurgence in popularity of these vehicles, it's not too difficult to find information that will guide you through basic repairs and maintenance. Since these are vehicles that are actually driven on the road regularly today, it's not too terribly hard to find spare parts, either.

Being able to handle repairs and find spare parts easily is a good thing because you will likely have to do this with frequency, unfortunately. Older vehicles, no matter how well maintained, are prone to breakdowns. Hoses wear out, parts get bent, you might run too hot or too cold, and things will simply stop working over time. If you choose an older vehicle like a Classic Van, try to get as complete a service history as possible. You might also luck out and find one with a new or refurbished engine, but always inspect all of the mechanical aspects — you never know when one of them is going to show their age.

Another consideration is the maintenance you can't handle on your own. Some of the older, foreign-built vehicles require special tools, parts, or mechanical knowledge. Rather than being able to breeze into any auto mechanic's garage, you will need to make sure someone on staff can repair your year, make, and model of van. A breakdown is always inconvenient, but extra frustrating when you have to spend time and energy figuring out where to go for assistance.

Additionally, things like "fuel efficiency" and "safety technology" are relatively new terms in the automotive world. Unlike today's vehicles, the vans of the 1960s didn't need to meet speed limits of 70 miles per hour regularly. Seatbelts didn't become mandatory until 1968. Airbags didn't become a requirement until 1998. Though Classic Vans are built like actual tanks in many regards, they are — by and large — lacking in the modern technology of current vehicles.

Conversion Vans

A Conversion Van is a type of van that is able to "convert" to a livable space. Early conversion vans of the 1970s simply added extra seating, or seats that folded into beds, and plush features, like carpeting and interior lighting. In the 1980s and 90s, features like televisions, VCRs, and indoor-style outlets were added to the category. Conversion vans are insulated, ventilated, and may be equipped with an isolated battery for a non-engine power source. In many ways, conversion vans are not unlike some of today's standard SUVs. But, even the most well-equipped conversion van will require some adaptation in order to be a full-time home.

Conversion vans are typically not too terribly expensive to purchase or maintain. It's relatively easy to find an older Chevy, Ford, or Dodge conversion van that has decent bones at a decent price. Since these vans are usually based on, very similar to, or completely identical to regular passenger vans, it's easy to find parts, and you won't need to find a mechanic who specializes in your particular van.

Spending less on the vehicle itself means you can allocate more funds toward the customization of the vehicle. It's also very likely that you'll find a Conversion Van that has some of the parts and pieces that you'll want in your finished van. For example, a lot of Conversion Vans have outward-swinging doors instead of sliding doors. Many manufacturers use this option as a way to stash fold-out tables or storage, which you can incorporate into your overall van scheme. Many also have built-in storage, which you can expand upon or leave as-is. You'll be able to enjoy seats with seatbelts that then fold into beds, saving you the problem of seats and beds as separate entities.

Some Conversion Vans were created with higher roofs, which may allow you to stand up comfortably but will definitely let you take advantage of more storage opportunities along the walls or roof.

Cargo Vans

Cargo Vans share the same advantages as Conversion Vans when it comes to being regularly maintained. Cargo Vans are being manufactured to this day, often as part of vehicle fleets for commercial and industrial businesses. Typically, Cargo Vans have a completely empty body, aside from a driver and passenger seat. Some have old tool racks, storage cabinets, or hanging storage in the back, depending on what they were used for in their past life. You may choose to incorporate or remove these to start fresh.

One thing that many Van Lifers enjoy about Cargo Vans is that they have very few windows. That means any wall is appropriate for building or storing. That also means you don't have to worry about looky-loos peeping in your van when it's parked or while you're sleeping.

On the flip side, both cargo and conversion vans typically have a lower fuel economy. While most options will function on regular unleaded gasoline, which tends to be less expensive, you will be stopping at fuel stations more regularly. You may also wish to keep spare fuel on hand for emergency situations.

You might find that many of the cargo vans on the market have very high mileage, especially if they were regularly used as part of a business. The advantage to this is that business vehicles are usually well-maintained since they're a crucial part of the operation. Still, you'll want to be prepared for any aging vehicle maintenance requirements that might come up.

Depending on your willingness to invest time and money into the van project, having no basic setup in a cargo van might also be a disadvantage. After all, you will need to create a liveable space out of nothing. You can find rehabbed cargo vans for sale, but these will cost more than a completely blank slate, of course. We'll talk more about what it takes to rehab and fully construct a living space in a van in the next chapter, but this is definitely something to keep in mind at this stage of the game, as well.

Euro Vans

First, bear in mind that the term "Euro Van" can refer to two different things. First, a Volkswagen Eurovan is a very specific make and model of van. These pop-top vans were offered in the US between 1993 and 2003, and many are still around and functional today.

There are others who refer to any European touring-style van as a "Euro Van." This can include Mercedes Sprinters, Klassen vans, Fiat Ducato, Renault Trafic, and other vehicles manufactured overseas. With the exception of the Mercedes Sprinter, it's not often you'll find these types of vans in the United States; however, with the growing market for off-grid options, more and more are arriving stateside.

When you're shopping for anything under the umbrella of "Euro Van," double-check if it's an actual VW Eurovan or a European van conversion.

Interestingly enough, VW Eurovans and Sprinter vans share a lot of common features. For example, they both are designed with large and small cargo storage options. They're more modern vehicles, which means you don't have to dredge up historical data to learn more about how they work. Additionally, as modern vehicles, they're equipped with smaller engines that are more powerful and consume less fuel.

Of course, there's a downside to this: as European creations, you'll need to find a mechanic who understands the engineering. They can also be difficult to find parts for, and expensive to repair. There will be more technical elements, such as computer systems, while the earlier and older models have more manual aspects.

Additionally, one thing to keep in mind about these taller vehicles is that you will need greater clearance. While this is typically not a problem on well-traveled highways, where semis and commuter buses are expected, this may pose a challenge on some of the more off-the-beaten-path locations you wish to visit. You can also encounter issues with parking garages if you find yourself within city limits.

Buses

There is a lot that can be said about buses, but the three basic options are School Bus, Coach, or Transit. Though the term "Skoolie" refers specifically to School Buses, the community as a whole tends to accept nearly any bus under the umbrella term.

There are significant differences between the three. True Skoolies are very affordable. Retired school buses can be acquired from multiple sources, including junkyard auctions, school district dispersal sales, online auctions, and more. There are several different lengths and configurations available as well.

Coach buses are bigger and bulkier than school buses, but they have one significant advantage: Uunder-cabin storage. If you've ever traveled the country by bus, you'll recall stowing your bags under the bus at the curb. This is great if you want to take along bicycles or large gear, or need to pack for all seasons. The size of the vehicle can be somewhat daunting though when navigating narrow city streets or winding mountain passages.

Transit buses are retired city buses. Like skoolies, these can come in various shapes and sizes. They rarely have the extra storage, but one unique feature is that some smaller city buses are equipped with wheelchair lifts or entry-assist options, which can be very helpful for those with mobility concerns.

Nearly all buses are equipped with a diesel engine, but some will have the engine in front, while others have the engine in the rear. If you're planning on running plumbing and electric wiring, you'll definitely need to mind the engine. You'll also need to know how to access it for repairs and maintenance, and pack the essential equipment, including any ladders or hydraulic lifts you might need.

One major downside to buses is that repair shops are extremely scarce for these vehicles. They tend to be pretty straightforward in their engineering, so it is possible to learn some DIY repair techniques, but if you're not mechanically inclined, you might have a rough time in the event of a breakdown.

Additionally, insurance can be a bit tricky on buses, but not impossible. As mentioned before, speak to your local representative to get the details before you go on a bus buying spree!

Campers
"Campers" is another somewhat ambiguous term. Some people call any van that you can sleep in a "camper." Others consider pull-behind trailers with living quarters "campers." For some, a "camper" is a full RV. Still others consider a "camper" a trailer that contains nothing more than room to sleep and adequate ventilation and weather protection.

There's a huge difference between an Airstream "camper" and a Patriot "camper" and a Vistabule "camper." When searching and shopping, be fully aware of what anything under the generic term "camper" entails.

For the most part, anything with the title of "camper" will be a prefabricated home on the road. It will include sleep areas, food prep areas, seating areas, and storage. There may be a bathroom, depending on the size of the camper. It may be a trailer instead of a combined living/driving space, such as in a van or a bus. Then again, one man's trailer is another man's camper!

When it comes to choosing the type of vehicle you plan to take on the road, there are really no "wrong" answers. While every class of vehicle has its own community that is completely devoted to that particular model, there are advantages and disadvantages to every single one. You'll find that even within these communities, there will be devotees to a certain year, make, or model.

Therefore, it's really impractical to listen to the recommendations of online forums, friends, or family members unless they face the same exact challenges, situations, and preferences as you will. Instead, pay attention to details. What are the dimensions? How many seats? What kind of engine does it have? What does its maintenance history look like? What type of fuel economy does it get? And most importantly — are you going to feel comfortable living in it?

Chapter 3: Ready-to-Roll, or Ready-to-Rehab?

The next consideration for your van home is how much work you want to put into transforming the space inside into the home of your dreams.

Ask yourself these two questions:

Do you want to create the ultimate space, in which you can comfortably live the rest of your life?

More importantly, are you willing to put in months or even years of hard work in order to create that space?

When asked what was most surprising about the process of gutting and rehabbing a van or bus, nearly everyone who has gone through the exercise will say the time of the entire process. When you browse those gorgeous van homes on the internet, see if you can't research the owners or builders to see how long they spent on the process. Many are very upfront with the process of refurnishing it, including all of the challenges that go along with that. After all, Van Life is a community effort!

Though many of the vans and skoolies you see on social media are labors of love, rebuilt from bare bones, you can start with a fully ready-to-roll vehicle. Yes, it will cost you more at the outset, but buying a fully rehabbed and refurbed vehicle means you won't have to strip the inside. You won't have to rewire anything. You won't have to learn practical plumbing. You won't have to create structures. You won't have to source lumber, nails, screws, tools, hinges... nothing! You can simply open the doors to your new home, look around, and decide where you want to put your belongings.

If that sounds like an absolute nightmare, then you are clearly more in the "Do It Yourself" camp. Before you purchase a giant transit bus and start demolition, there are a few things you need to ask yourself:

How much time can you devote each day to construction?
For many, construction starts out as a "little bit each day" type of project, but swiftly becomes a full obsession. There will be setbacks. Things will not work out exactly as planned. You will cut a piece of insulation multiple times, trying to get it to fit along a curved wall... and eventually, you will cut it to the point where you can't use it. You will find that the plumbing absolutely cannot go there, or there, or really anywhere that it might make sense. Every person who has ever changed anything about their van has been in this exact position.

And that is how we become obsessed — this drive to solve all problems immediately takes over all reason. At the same time, you might still be working your day job as you work on your van space. Your partner, your children, your dog and cat, might all be rightfully concerned that you're spending all night in the van.

This is an easy way to burn yourself out on the whole project. As you encounter one frustration after another, you might decide it's not worth it. While we have no practical cures for the difficulties you'll no doubt encounter, it is highly recommended that you work on your van or bus slowly and surely, rather than trying to rush through it. If you're planning a very extensive makeover, don't plan to leave in two months.
A simple rule of thumb: If time is of the essence, choose something that's ready to go (or at least very close). If you want to really create something from the ground up, don't have a deadline.

Can You Build It?

Be very honest with yourself: do you know anything about construction, electricity, plumbing, insulation, drywall, cabinetry, etc.? Or, are you handy enough that you feel very confident about learning? Can you see a straight line, take a variety of accurate measurements, and execute the product in your mind?

There are four main steps to the process of creating your dream space inside a van.

First, you need to gut it. This is especially true if you purchase a bus that still has the seats inside. You will need to remove everything, and you will need to somehow get rid of it or repurpose it.

As a side note, you will need to be creative when it comes to the collection of school bus seats you're about to have if you've gone with a skoolie. Some folks have luck selling them "as is" to people in the area or via online auctions. More likely, you'll want to take them apart and sell the metal for scrap. Unless you have loads of space in which to store dozens of seats, this is something you ought to plan on doing before you bring your skoolie home, too.

Once you've got your open space, you need a functional design. You'll need to consider not just the overall flow, but where you're going to put the heaviest weight loads, where you're going to put storage or built-ins, and the reality of where you can put plumbing or electricity, which might be based on where you put the water source or hook up, generator, or solar panels. You'll need to be aware of where and how the doors open, as well as the windows.

Most people who have completely gutted and refurbished a van report having at least two to three versions of their design plans, so don't be too concerned if your first plan has to be scrapped. Learn, and move on.

Next comes executing the design. You'll need to run any electric and plumbing before you put in insulation and walls. You'll have to put in walls before you build structures, such as cabinets, seating areas, or sleeping areas.

A side note about storage: One of the best ways to maximize storage is to put it under seating or sleeping areas. One very popular trick is to raise the sleeping area as high as you can, to create a larger storage space beneath. You can build the frame of your bed over a cabinet system to create both open and closed storage underneath your bed. Perhaps you add a fold-out table to the base of your bed or seating that pulls out like a drawer. The options are infinite!

As you are constructing your new home, you will need both materials and tools. Of the two, the tools might be the most cost-prohibitive, as well as the hardest to source. You will also make multiple trips to the hardware store each week. Therefore, you must account in your budget for tools, supplies, as well as gas money and time spent at the hardware store acquiring these things. You might see if there is a tool-lending program in your community, as this can save you several hundred dollars. You might also cruise local selling walls to see if there are used tools available in your area. The unfortunate truth about these processes though, is that you might not find what you need exactly when you need it.

Despite all of your best intentions, there will be waste. Anything from bent nails to stripped screws, to perfectly usable lumber cut to the wrong length. You will not want to keep this waste forever, so consider a plan that will allow you to collect, remove, and appropriately dispose of it. This may mean a call to a junkyard or working with your regular waste management company.

Can You Afford It?

The cost figures for fully renovating a skoolie range from $10,000 to $30,000. Granted, that's cost over time, and as mentioned earlier, it can take years to fully construct the space of your dreams.

We've alluded to some of the expenses here, but let's put it all on the table.

You'll need:

- tools
- safety equipment, such as goggles and gloves
- lumber
- screws, nails, hinges, knobs, sliding rails, bolts, and anchors
- wiring
- insulation
- plugs and switches
- pipes
- walls
- countertops/ sealed surfaces
- flooring
- faucets and fixtures for water closet

This doesn't include any decorative items, such as backsplashes or paint, or power and water supplies, which we'll discuss in more detail in the next chapter. It also doesn't include any books, courses, or instruction you might pay for to help you with your endeavors.

Do You Have the Work Space?

If you're going to be working on a vehicle for months or years, you need a space where you can safely and legally do so.

It is unlikely that a skoolie will fit in the garage of your suburban home. It is also unlikely that you'll be permitted to work extensively on demo and rehab in the parking garage of a city condo building. If you know someone who has a large yard where you can work, that might be a great option... until the neighbors call the city.

There are legal considerations for working on vehicles within some city or corporation limits. Even if you're not disposing of harmful liquids, less enthusiastic neighbors might consider your activities a nuisance. Therefore, you'll want to find a nice, large space — preferably indoors — where you can work on your vehicle. And then a backup location. And possibly even a backup to the backup. Whether you wear out your welcome or simply outgrow your space, you'll need a plan, since you can't just plop a large bus or very tall van down anywhere.

Most beginner van projects are somewhere in between "completely ready" and "completely reconstructed." You might choose a "mostly ready" van, and lift the bed to add storage or shorten the sleeping area to add a food prep area. You might start with only the minimal changes, then add a little room here or include a fold-out table there as you spend time living in your new space.

Alternatively, you might feel that life on the road is not complete unless you have a wood-burning stove, fully functional skylights, and a hand-painted porcelain backsplash in the bathroom. There's nothing wrong with this perspective, either.

Ultimately, creating your van space is a balance between what you *want* to do, and what you *can* do. If there is a significant overlap between the two, then best wishes on your rehab and refurb experience! If you find that you're lacking in time, skill, funds, or space, you might scale back your project. You might wish to find a mostly-ready van or add the assistance of a professional if the issue is time or skill.

The internet is full of experiences shared by those who have made this journey before. We'll share a few links in the **resources guide** to get you started. When it comes to the building stage, however, you truly cannot research too much, especially if you are a novice DIY-er. You'll want to consider safety, practicality, usability, and durability of everything you construct to be 100% sure before you lay the first nail or cut the first board!

And most of all, have patience and faith. Whether or not it turns out exactly as you dreamed, it will turn out exactly as you have built it. Your planning and patience will pay off in the end.

Chapter 4: Budget Considerations for Creating Your Van

While it may seem that we harp and harp on the concept of budget, you'll find that this is with good reason. One of the most common reasons people give up on the van life dream is because they run out of money before they even have the chance to hit the road.

While it's true that you can save quite a bit of money by abandoning regular bills, multiple car payments, mortgages, and the like with the vagabond lifestyle of the road, you will need to invest a bit of money into setting up the lifestyle to be sustainable.

For those who feel cooped up, you might be so passionately drawn to the experience that you feel like you could simply hop in any old van and drive off and "make it work." There is a very specific demographic for whom this is true. If you have plenty of money, the ability to take on any odd jobs no matter where you are, no particular preference about where you sleep at night, a decent cooler, and a reliable propane burner, then it is possible to "make it work."

If you have a family, pets, the desire to have a predictable shower and bathroom experience, the ability to prepare a variety of fresh foods, and the need to sleep in a comfortable bed, then you will need to plan very carefully in the early stages.

So, when it comes to budgeting, we started at the overall "big picture" of all of the various categories of expenses that might come into play. Now it's time to start drilling down into more detail, starting with the van itself.

How Much Will It Cost to Hit the Road?

The equation for determining the overall cost of your van is as follows:

Cost of Vehicle + Cost of Repairs/Rehab/Refurb = Pre-Road Cost

(Cost of oil/oil change x 6) + cost of tires + cost for replacement cost + hourly rate for emergency maintenance = Annual Upkeep Cost

Size of fuel tank x Average Miles Per Gallon = Miles Per Tank
Total Distance Traveled (divided by) Miles Per Tank = Total Number of Fuel Stops
(Size of fuel tank x going rate for fuel) x Number of Fuel Stops = Total Fuel Budget

Pre-Road Cost + Annual Upkeep Cost + Total Fuel Budget is the amount you will need to get you through the first year on the road.

There are ways to maximize your money, however.

First, remember that the bigger the vehicle, the more fuel it will need. Consider purchasing the smallest possible van or bus that you can actually live in. This might require you to do the "try it at home" test a few times with different configurations.

In addition, consider planning your wandering strategically. Instead of California one week and Connecticut the next, consider taking some time to wind along the West Coast. Try finding a good central location where you can park for a longer period of time, and use a bicycle or small motorbike or scooter to explore the sights nearby. This will not only save fuel costs but wear and tear costs on your van as a whole, minimizing maintenance costs. Lastly, if you find a free spot to camp within National Lands, you'll save a significant amount of money on camp fees and site fees while you do this exploration. Another thing to keep in mind when looking at the annual budget is your income. We'll discuss working from the road in more detail shortly, but there are ways to make money while you travel. Any income you make will offset your expenses, of course, and can either go toward regular maintenance and fuel or toward an emergency fund.

Power and Water: The Utilities

There are also some features you can add to the van construction that will help you save, as well. If you add a power supply and water supply, you'll have a fully self-sustaining home on wheels. This means you'll have a lower reliance on stopping at full-service camping parks. You'll be able to produce the power to charge your phones and devices, as well as have a functioning bathroom to help with showers and general clean up.

When it comes to power supplies, the top two options are generators and solar power. Each option has, of course, strong arguments for and against them.

First, let's look at generators:

Pros	Cons
Produce a lot of instant power at any time	Noisy
Not weather dependent	Require fuel and ongoing maintenance
Can handle a lot of wattage	May be prohibited in some locations due to fumes

Now let's look at the argument surrounding solar power:

Pros	Cons
No fumes, no noise, no maintenance	Does not create a lot of power
Can be repositioned as necessary	Power supply is dependent upon intake/positioning
No on-going expenses: install and done	Can be damaged, which requires replacement

All said, it boils down to your personal preference and budget. A generator will be an ongoing expense but will be able to supply great quantities of instant power. This might be a greater advantage than disadvantage if you're going to need to power a laptop, phone, and WiFi hotspot. On the other hand, if you won't need tons of power all the time, solar panels might be a real budget-saving option.

There are Van Lifers who live without power. You can choose this route as well. Between independent battery charge units, USB plugs in more modern vehicles, and the old-fashioned type of plug that uses a decommissioned cigarette lighter port, it's possible to keep a cell phone charged. You can also take breaks at fast food restaurants, rest stations, or laundromats, and mooch a little power while you fuel your own body, shower, or catch up on some laundry. Before you help yourself to some power, make sure it's allowed. It also probably goes without saying, but never leave your phone unattended, as it will very likely take a voyage of its own. And if you're going to borrow a little electricity, it's considered good road manners if you make a purchase while you're there.

The next consideration is the water supply. If you are going to carry your own water supply, you'll need two tanks — one for freshwater, and one for greywater. Most experts recommend each tank hold up to 5-7 gallons. The main factor in deciding how big of a tank you want is how much you can carry yourself, as you'll be responsible for filling, maintaining, and emptying these tanks. One gallon of water weighs approximately 8 pounds, for reference. Therefore, a five-gallon tank will be a heft of close to 50 pounds, once you include the weight of the tank itself.

You'll also want to make sure that any tank, pipes, or tubing involved with your freshwater supply is FDA-rated as food safe.

Greywater tanks do not have to be food-safe, but are just as important. "Greywater" refers to wastewater from your sink, shower, etc.

You'll want to make sure that both your freshwater and greywater tanks are both accessible and secured, so they are equally available for filling and emptying, and don't slosh around while you drive.

If you're looking for a very simple way to access freshwater, consider the gravity method. This basically involves installing the water supply in a way that gravity delivers the water through the tubing, to your waiting hands, cup, bucket, or wherever you need the water to go. Many rudimentary van shower systems use this method by hanging the water supply over a door or from an overhead hook, and releasing a valve so the water flows freely.

For those who wish to have more control over water flow, a manual hand or foot pump can be installed. Hand pumps require very little mechanical know-how and involve a temporary or fixed pump being added to the open end of the freshwater tank. The design is not unlike a soap or lotion bottle pump dispenser, only on a larger scale. Foot pumps will require a directed flow via a faucet and sink so that the greywater tank catches the runoff and waste, but they offer excellent control over how much water is dispensed at a time.

Lastly, there's the option of an electric water pump. For this option, you will likely prefer a generator that you can run at least part-time to assist with the process, as you'll need at least 12 volts of electricity. With this choice, you do have the option to install a water heater so that you'll have continuous hot water, as well. You can also add an accumulator, which will store a little water each time the water is turned on. The accumulator will let you use a bit of water even when the power is off, which will save on noise and expense.

Then there's the toilet. Technology has come a long way in this regard, so your van won't have to be as primitive as you fear... unless, of course, you want it that way. There are a variety of road-ready commodes available that can be incorporated into your new abode with or without plumbing.

First, there are composting toilets. These toilets are chemical-free and store your waste until you can dispose of it. The secret is a peat mixture and a dehydration process. The liquids go into a separate bottle, which can be dumped securely, while the solids mix with the peat and turn into safe compost. These toilets do require power in order to work, however, as most include a small fan that keeps the process working. Composting toilets can be very expensive, but a very wise investment for those who wish to use the toilet indoors with the most minimal need for chemicals, hassle, or interacting with the resulting matter.

Then there are portable potties. These are small, self-contained toilet units that can be installed anywhere. They feature a waste tank and a water tank and can be "flushed" like a standard toilet, although what's flushed will await future disposal in the appropriate tank. This means that chemicals should be used to keep odor at bay between emptyings, though eco-friendly chemicals are also readily available. These toilets do use a considerable amount of water and can get heavy depending on how long you go between emptying.

Those traveling with children or in groups may want to invest in a full electric camper-style toilet. While impractical to install on a smaller van, this format is suitable for buses, where a waste tank can be stashed under the vehicle and dumped appropriately in waste stations at campgrounds. The benefit here is that you don't have an immediate or urgent worry about overflow, no possible spillage, and the toilet is a permanent part of your home. The downside is that it will have to be incorporated and installed, thus taking up valuable space and requiring a sizable investment.

There are also a variety of low-tech options. From what amounts to a stool with no seat, to a bucket with a seat on it, many Van Lifers have made the most of an awkward situation with a practical — if not at all glamorous — solution. There are multiple small battery-operated or hand-pump style toilets on the market as well, but bear in mind, these are often very low to the ground and still require regular and frequent emptying. Also, consider the fact that you may need to use this device at any hour of the day, in all kinds of weather. Make sure you choose a toilet option that you'll feel comfortable with at midnight during a thunderstorm!

It is possible to live without any plumbing whatsoever, of course. Water can be found in many places, and it's very simple to stock up on gallons of usable drinking water. This will, however, require room for storage. A cooler is a multi-level solution when it comes to water usage, as well. The ice used to keep food fresh in a cooler will, over time, melt. While you might not want to use that water for drinking, you can heat it up with your propane burner and a pot, and enjoy a bath or shower. You can also use that melted ice water to cool off when temperatures are climbing. Toilets can be found at gas stations, restaurants, grocery stores, campgrounds, parks, and rest areas.

When disposing of greywater and waste, it is crucial that you do not contaminate any water sources. Make sure you only dump wastewater in approved and appropriate areas. Composting toilets are less dodgy since the waste has been decontaminated naturally, but some toilet solutions include chemicals that can poison humans and wildlife, and destroy native plants and soil. Whenever possible, use biodegradable, environmentally friendly soaps, cleaners, and toilet papers.

If you choose to go the "natural" route, remember to be courteous. Step away from main areas — even if you're camping on free land, you can still avoid areas where people are likely to walk. Dig your waste trench at least six inches deep, and be sure to bury everything thoroughly once you're done.

Chapter 5: The Search Process

Once you've got all of your plans in hand, it's time to make them so. You know what size vehicle you need and likely have a top-three selection of the type of vehicle you'd like to purchase. You are confident about what you want to put in your van or bus, where it's going to go, and what you need to do to make it happen.

Now stack all of those plans neatly, and throw everything on the floor except your budget.

Shopping for your van or bus or camper can be agonizing if you have very specific requirements. You may choose to wait until you are able to locate The Exact Perfect Vehicle for your adventure. Alternatively, you may choose something that is more of a compromise on your exact requests but meets all your requirements. The choice is entirely your own.

The internet is a fantastic place to find Van Life resources. As a community that has no physical footprint (or rather, one that is always in motion), there are many forums and sites where van dwellers meet up to share thoughts, ideas, and ask each other questions. In fact, we've included some of these in the **resource section** of this book.

As you read through these forums, you'll find discussions about particular types of vans or skoolies, as well as sales ads. Some people within the van community make a fair living off rehabbing and selling vehicles. Others find that they "outgrow" their van and are ready to step up to a bigger, more off-road capable, or in some cases, more frugal vehicle.

Another online resource is vehicle sales sites. Again, we've compiled a few suggestions to get you started in the **resource section**. There are sites dedicated to vans and buses, but you can also find some good deals on regular automotive sites, especially if you're looking for a cargo or conversion van that you can take down to the bare floor and remodel into your own.

There is some debate as to whether it's worth it to reach out to regular car dealerships. The answer is yes. Shopping for a van is not unlike shopping for any other specialty item, like antique glass or rare book printings. You never know where they're going to turn up. You might find just the right base vehicle has come into a dealership as a trade-in and swipe it up before they list it on an online auction. One benefit to this plan is that dealers seldom let vehicles leave their lot without at least a full inspection. Though they might not take the time, or invest the money into fixing anything that's out of sorts, they'll at least be aware and disclose this information to you. Auctions are another great resource, if you're ok with buying vehicles "as is." You might not know its issues, problems, or need for repairs until you get it home and start truly inspecting it, but the vehicle you purchase at an auction can be extremely cheap.

Online auctions have similar perils — you are relying on the word of the person selling the vehicle, and you may not be able to physically inspect the vehicle until you have already paid for it. Still, online auction sites can bring great luck to those who have done their homework and are ready for just about anything.

If you're specifically looking for a bus, you can reach out directly to the source for more information about obtaining one of their decommissioned vehicles. For skoolies, you can reach out to the school district. Frequently, their vehicles pass through local auto auctions, but it's possible the school district might be interested in making a deal, for the right price.

When it comes to coach-type buses, you might need to do a bit more digging. National bus lines will have a point of contact for decommissioned buses, but if you're dealing with a more local outfit, it might require a few calls and emails before you find the right person.

The city transit department will likely have information about what happens to city buses once they're removed from duty. In many cases, they end up in junkyards, auctions, or are donated to various programs, but again, you might be able to make arrangements for purchase first.

When it comes to pulling the trigger and purchasing your vehicle, you must feel fully confident in your decision. You must have addressed all budget considerations, all repair requirements, and be ready to shoulder the burden of any rehab and remodeling that will be needed to make your van or bus your new home.
We encourage everyone to do as much research as possible. Find a

handful of options. Decide what things you can compromise on and what features are absolute necessities. Can you wiggle on price? What if you find a vehicle that has higher mileage than you'd like, but the price is perfect, and it's been well-cared for? It is highly unlikely that you'll find a vehicle that meets all of your needs precisely. What is far more likely is that you'll find a vehicle that shows you what features, options, and qualities are really most important to you.

If it is at all possible, try to test drive the vehicle. This might mean doing some traveling. Worse yet — this might mean getting your hopes up, traveling, and discovering it's not going to work.

You will have to feel comfortable driving your new home. In the case of a larger bus, it will take time before driving such a massive vehicle feels natural, but if a simple trip around the block feels desperately uncomfortable for any reason, it might be a good time to head back to the drawing board. There are things that can be altered, improved, or modified, but if you decide you really don't like the way driving a van with a manual transmission feels, it might be less expensive to check out options with an automatic transmission, rather than replace the entire system.

You'll also want the opportunity to really inspect the vehicle in detail. This means you might have to take a crash course in the year, make, and model of the vehicle you're going to check out, but it's better to be fully informed than guessing.

Additionally, see what maintenance and repair records you can get your hands on. The more you know about this particular vehicle's history, the more you can plan for future issues — or at least identify what needs your immediate attention.

Advice from the Road- Part 2

When it came to purchasing our first van, I was adamant that it would have a kitchenette, or at least a purposed food-prep area with storage and running water. My plans for the interior included a fold-out table, which I could use as a work station during the day, and could do extra duty as an eating surface, a drying rack for dishes and laundry, or a spot where we could hang out and play games or plan the next leg of our voyage.

I wanted an automatic transmission. I wanted a vehicle no more than 25 years old. I was fine with higher mileage, as long as it was well-cared for and didn't come with any major problems. I didn't care about color, and I wasn't fussy about how the sleeping area was set up.

We ended up with a VW Vanagon from the 1980s. It did not have a kitchen area. It didn't have a fold-out table. It didn't have so much as a shelf. In the back was a platform and a mattress... that's it.

Instead, it had a recently replaced engine. It had been regularly serviced for the past 30 years. It had only had two owners and still had its original owner's manual (which is roughly the same size as a 1980s phone book, by the way). It came with a automatic transmission, as he hoped, and a gaudy peace sign sticker... which actually hid a deep ding in the side of the door.

Was it the van I had planned on purchasing? Absolutely not. Was I completely wooed by its mechanical soundness, ease of operation, and blank-slate space? Very much so.

We looked at several dozen vans. Some of them we just courted online until the inevitable Huge Issue came to light. We had the chance to kick some of the tires. But when we found this van, two states away, in a heated, climate-controlled garage, I knew that this was the main contender for our future home on wheels.

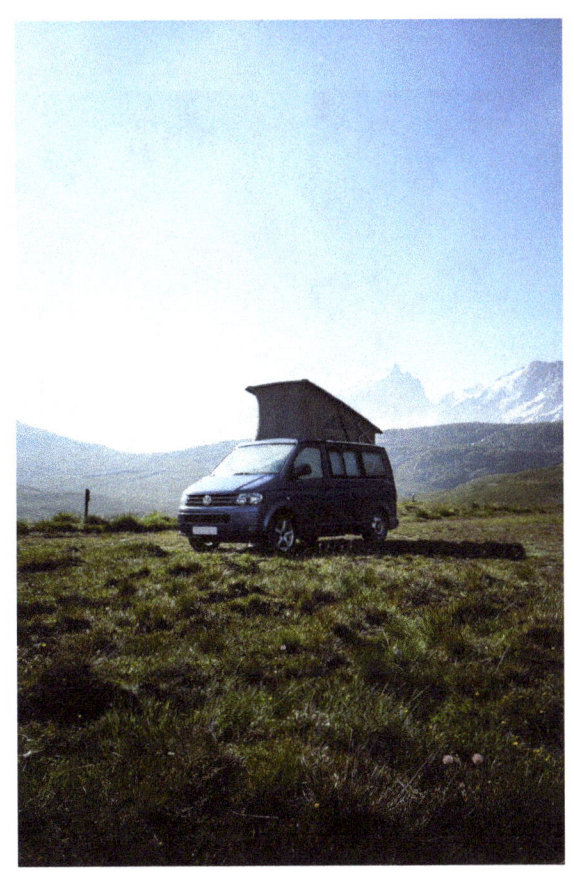

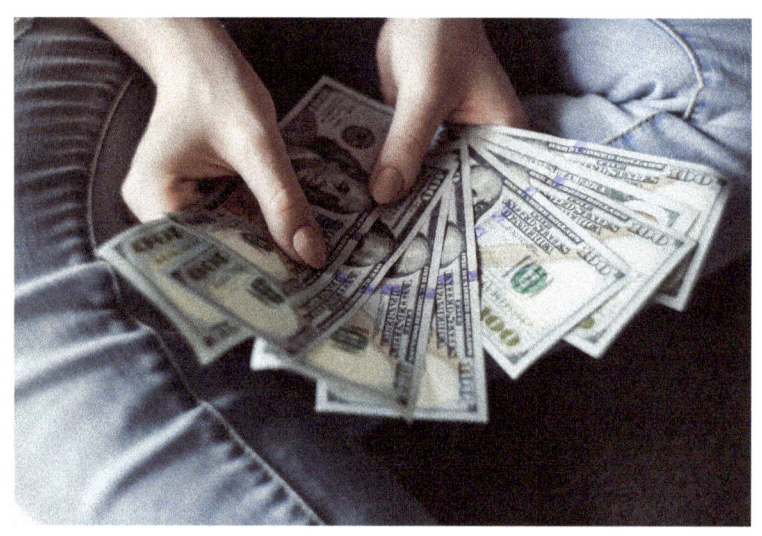

Section 3: Creating and Maintaining a Budget While on the Road

There are so many factors that go into both creating and maintaining a budget while you're on the road. Here we'll attempt to walk through the process in easy-to-handle pieces.

If you've even started considering your Van Life budget, your head is probably a whirlwind of figures, with questions like:

1. What can I afford to spend each month?
2. What splurges or luxury items will I allow myself?
3. What happens if I run out of money?
4. If I buy this item now, will it cost me more or less in the long run?
5. What'll I do in an emergency? (Followed by feelings of desperation and panic, usually.)

First, take a deep breath. Having an emergency while on the road is really no different than having an emergency at any other time of your life. You can't completely prepare for everything, and while it's going to be deeply inconvenient, you'll have to take everything step by step to move in the right direction.

As for the rest of the questions, we'll address them one by one. While we can't actually sit down with you and do the math for your particular situation, we can bring you some key points and advice from folks who have been on the road, to help you decide where to spend money, where to save money, and where to make money.

Advice from the Road: Part 3
When we first took our van out, we had nothing. Ok, that's not entirely true. We had a bed, tons of really intuitive storage, a large ice-vault type cooler with a valve on the side to empty out the water, and a propane burner with two fuel tanks. Our van didn't even have interior lights until we removed the non-functioning air conditioning unit and accidentally reconnected something.

We thought this was the best way to save money — live as basically and frugally as possible, right? Barebones means no waste, little investment, and a smaller budget. Well, it turns out that we accidentally sabotaged ourselves with this mindset.

We stocked up on what we considered "van food" beforehand. As experienced campers and hikers, we assumed we'd want to eat the same sort of thing in the van that we ate while camping. We thought we were brilliant.

Well, it turns out that, when you're parked in a camp park full of families grilling huge, juicy steaks, that dehydrated chicken curry packet doesn't look so appetizing anymore. Even worse, because your home has wheels, and because you can get an internet signal nearly anywhere, it is very, very tempting to find yourself at the local famous restaurant every night. Which would you prefer: a powdered camping meal or authentic mole enchiladas served by a woman who has her family's 300-year-old recipe?

It's easy to make excuses, too. After all, you're on the road to experience the world as it is, and that includes the local flavor — literally. Problem is, eating at restaurants eats your budget right up!

So, you learn to compromise. Head to local markets and grocery stores, and stock up on local products there. We could buy all the flavors we couldn't find at home and take them with us wherever we went.

We did have to change the cooler setup, though. We thought we were being budget-conscious by getting the less expensive cooler. Unfortunately, we ended up wasting a lot of food when it got "drowned" in the melting ice.

As a result, we had to modify our entire setup. Just for food? No — to make the most out of our budget. Our no-power, no-water setup was tweaked into a solution that actually reduced our spending. We use only three 160-watt solar panels, which connect to four batteries. These also keep us working while we're on the road. We no longer have to stop at cafes or restaurants and buy something for the privilege of "borrowing" electricity and WiFi — we're self-reliant. (Think about it — even if you just buy a $3 snack each day for an hour of guilt-free power, that's $90 a month, and that's with a very low estimate!)

Even better, we have far less food waste. We invested in a more expensive cooler, which plugs into the van's cigarette lighter socket while we're on the road and can connect with the solar battery converter when we're not in motion. Just in case, we have several cooler packs that don't leak, spill, or otherwise ruin our food. We also have a full series of BPA-free food storage containers of all sizes, so if we do need to temporarily run on ice, we lose nothing.

Do we still try out local cuisine at restaurants? Sure, from time to time. But choosing to be able to store and prepare our own fresh food is a decision that required a little more spending on the front end but has saved us literally thousands of dollars each month!

Chapter 1: Determining Your Budget

At its core, a budget is simply a balance between money you have and money you need (or want) to spend. When you live in a fixed, permanent location, it's pretty easy to see what you have, what you need, and what to expect from month to month. After all, our daily routines rarely change overall — and that's why the road is calling to you!

Still, there's something to be said for predictability. Most of us rest easier with at least some perceived control over our daily, weekly, and monthly expenses.

It may feel, at first, like heading out on the road is going to be a complete upheaval of your way of life. In many ways, this is true. But there are plenty of things that aren't going to change about your lifestyle. You'll still need to eat every day. You'll still need to drink plenty of water. You'll still have dirty laundry.

We've included a chart that includes some common ongoing expenses. Bear in mind that this chart only includes expenses that you'll encounter on a continuous basis—we'll get to the start up and packing expenses in a moment.

This is, of course, just a guide to get you started. If you have children on the trip, some of these categories might change a bit. The maintenance for any equipment you install, such as toilets, generators, hot water heaters, and such, will be dependent on what type of equipment you choose and its specific requirements. If you have a pet, you'll need to take their needs into consideration. However, this chart should get you started in the process of thinking about what you need on a running basis.

Expense Category	Considerations	Your Calculation
Fuel	Price per Gallon Miles per Gallon Distance Traveled Fuel Cost Fluctuations (by location) Emergency Fuel Supply	
Maintenance	Oil changes (5-10,000 miles) Tire rotation (5-7,000 miles) Air filter Fluids (Radiator, Transmission, Coolant, Brake, Air Conditioning, Washer, Power Steering) Glass Cracks Windshield Wiper Blades	
Location	Parking pass Camping pass Park entry fees Showers Hotels (if necessary) Greywater dump fees (charged at some campsites)	
Kitchen Supplies	Drinking water Food/Groceries Cleaning tools	

Health	Toiletries (shampoo, toothpaste, soap, etc.) Vitamins Medications (both prescription and OTC) First Aid supplies (bandages, antiseptic cream, cotton swabs) Sunscreen Bug spray Regular medical check-ups, vaccines, dental care
Laundry	Detergent Laundromat costs
Entertainment	Entry fees Park passes Restaurants Cafes/Wineries/Breweries/Distilleries/etc. Gifts/games/toys
Other ongoing expenses	Insurance (Medical, Vehicle, etc.) Generator upkeep (if used) Vet bills (if you bring a pet) Credit card bills Van payment (if you take out a loan for the van) Roadside Assistance Program Cell phone bill WiFi
Expenses from Home (applies only if you choose to maintain your home while you're on the road)	Mortgage/rent Electric/gas/water House sitter/tenant Insurance Taxes

When you're filling out these expenses, try to be both practical and generous in your estimates. No matter where you're traveling, the cost of living is largely based on location. A gallon of water that costs 60 cents at one grocery store might cost $1.09 at another store twenty miles away. You can shop around for bargains, but that might cut into your fuel budget. Unless you're able to really sit down and cruise the internet to find deals at local stores and any relevant coupons, try to plan things out.

You might notice that we included "expenses from home." For some van dwellers, it's impossible to break a lease or sell property in time to get on the road. Some actually maintain their homes, so they have a "base" to return to from time to time. They might have a tenant renting the home or sublease an apartment. If you choose to maintain a stationary home, there will be expenses associated with that location — a mortgage in your name, bills, etc. You'll definitely not want any unpleasant financial surprises while you're on the road, so be sure that you factor in those regular payments if you will have them.

There are also things you can stock up on beforehand, to some extent and expenses that you will only encounter at the start of your trip, and perhaps rarely afterward. Let's take a look at what those might look like.

Expense Category	Considerations	Your Calculation
Emergency Supplies	Storage bin Tarps Bungee cords Duct tape Road flares Jumper cables Tire patch kit Spare gas canister Jack Tool kit	
Camping/Outdoor Supplies	Storage bin Tent/equipment Backpacks Sleeping bags Flashlights/lanterns Batteries Multi-tool	
Health and Wellness	Mirror Tote for toiletries Scissors Towels Storage for dirty laundry	
Bedding	Pillows Sheets Variety of blankets Mattress/sleeping surface Storage for unused bedding	

Kitchen	Large container to store canned/boxed/dry food
	Cooler or refrigerator
	Small containers for open food/leftovers
	Pots and pans
	Cooking tools (spatula, serving spoons, can opener, bottle opener)
	Eating utensils
	Dishes
	Burner or stovetop
	Fuel for cooktop
	Dish bin
	Dishrags

Again, this is not a comprehensive list for every possible scenario, but a few helpful guidelines to get you thinking about what items are part of your necessary routine.

Many of these items will need to be replaced depending on the length of your trip, and in case there is any accidental damage. Overall these will not be things that need to be replaced weekly or even monthly.

Advice from the Road: Part 4
A word about storage.

Everything in your van will need a place to live. Everything.

One of the most challenging parts of living in a van is the fact that you can't put your dirty laundry on a chair and deal with it on laundry day. You can't just let the dishes hang out overnight in the sink. Your van will become very crowded, messy, stinky, and full of pests unless you stash your dirty laundry somewhere, keep your dishes clean and put away, and your surfaces tidy.

Worse yet, if you leave food sitting out, you run the risk of attracting bears, coyote, wolves, and more. While not naturally aggressive, these critters are very interested in any tasty tidbits you might have onboard, and they're naturally equipped with the claws and jaws that will help them get what they want!

When we hit the road, we started with several large bins:

- *One for our emergency supplies, which we labeled the Oh S**t Kit*
- *One for the kitchen goods, which included dry foods and all of our kitchenwares*
- *One for our camping gear, so if it got wet or muddy, it wouldn't roll all over the van and make a mess*
- *One for our dirty laundry — trust me, you want something that seals, especially if you're going to be hiking ten miles a day!*

These were each 60 gallon "under the bed box"-style heavy duty bins with lockable lids, specifically chosen to fit under the sleeping area. We could reach under the bed at any time and slide out the bin we needed — which we could identify because they were labeled on all four sides. The labels weren't anything fancy; just a strip of duct tape with the "Kitchen," "Camp," and so on written in permanent marker.

Under the shelf where these large bins lived was a storage area accessed by smaller doors. This had been where the original owner stored his emergency kit. We chose to create 6-quart sized plastic bins with lids to place in this area. They fit perfectly through the small door, and that way, wouldn't roll around or require additional containment.

We each had two — I chose to make one my toiletry kit — I put my shampoo, conditioner, soap, toothpaste, toothbrush, and hairbrush in one bin. That way, whenever we stopped at a place that had showers or ran into a rest stop to brush our teeth and wash our faces, I didn't have to pick and juggle what I needed — just grab the box and go. And since it had a lid, I didn't have to worry about things falling out and getting lost. If you've ever had a toothbrush fall on a rest area floor, you know that sinking feeling in your stomach when you lose an important piece of equipment!

My second bin held what I considered my daily necessities: medication, a spare phone charger, hair ties, the muscle rub I put on at night, dry *shampoo, hand lotion, lip balm, sunburn cream, and my mobile TENS unit. I also had a small bottle of air freshener in there, for that "we really need to make today laundry day" vibe.*

When it comes to living in a van, space is at a premium. You don't want things rolling around while you're driving, and you don't want to search all over the place when you're looking for something. If you can create a storage solution for every major area of your daily life, you'll make life so much easier for yourself.

You just have to remember to put everything back where you found it!

Chapter 2: Sticking to It

Now that you have an idea of what your expenses are going to look like, you've got to put some guidelines in place to help you stick to this plan. You know yourself best of all, so if you feel like there will be some moments of excess — such as visiting your favorite theme park or splurging at a restaurant you've always wanted to visit — make sure you add these into your budget at the outset. Just like when you lived in a stationary home, you want to make sure you have as much control over your money as possible.

There are many things you can do to keep your budget low, but you'll have to do some research and planning to carry out these options.

For example, making your own food is going to be considerably less expensive than eating at restaurants several times a week. But, as mentioned in Advice from the Road: Part 3, you'll need to be adequately prepared. Living on ramen every night is neither enjoyable nor nutritious. Make sure you incorporate methods for storing canned, boxed, and dry food, as well as produce, proteins, juices, leftovers, and other things that need to be kept chilled. This way, you'll be able to create healthful, tempting, budget-friendly meals without wasting food. We'll provide some tips on this topic in a later chapter.

Another place where you can save loads of money is by scouting out free parking and camping. Your online van community is possibly the best resource for finding a free place to catch some rest with travelers sharing some of their favorite spots for anyone who is currently on the road.

While there is nothing wrong with pulling into a paid campsite for the night, it can start to eat away at your budget. Many campsites require a $20-$40 per night camping fee, and if they have any extra perks, like vault toilets, WiFi, electricity, water hookups, laundry, or showers, there might be an additional fee to use those services.

Whenever possible, consider finding free camping. In the United States, National forests and wildlife areas and land owned by the Bureau of Land Management, they welcome free camping — as long as the land isn't privately owned. You'll need to do your homework in order to discover these spots, however, and there are several areas where there simply aren't public lands. We've included a few links in the **resource section** to guide your search.

Staying Green is another way to keep expenses down. This includes things like choosing reusable rags over paper products. Using as little water as possible for cleaning and reusing your greywater in practical ways or other options. If you use a generator, consider running it as little as possible. Try solar-powered flashlights — they can charge in the sunshine on your dashboard during the day and light up the van at night. If you don't need to be in motion, stay parked.

Anything you can do yourself saves you an expense, too. This includes maintenance and repair of nearly everything that's in your van or skoolie. If you can learn to perform minor mechanical repairs, you'll only need to pay for parts. If you can repair your own clothing, you won't need to replace it. If you have a roof rack and a sunny day, perhaps you save your quarters on a dryer and air dry your laundry.

Lastly, it's not a bad idea to sign up for fuel perks or discount programs, especially at national chains. Fuel is going to be a constant expense, and if you have the ability to earn discounts, you'll certainly be able to take advantage of them. You might also choose a credit card program through a gas station that provides discounts on fuels and products purchased from that chain. You may also stock up on gift cards for particular gas stations — some of them offer heavy discounts if you purchase gift cards in bulk. Investigate all of your opportunities to save on fuel, since you'll have absolutely no way of predicting what a gallon of gas will cost from one day to another!

Chapter 3: Earning Income While on the Move

If Van Life is to become your full-time lifestyle, you'll need either a very large amount of money before you hit the road, or you'll need regular income. More and more van dwellers are choosing to work while they're on the move. This can take on many shapes.

1. After completely rehabbing and rebuilding a van, you might find you're rather handy. Whenever money runs low, you go into a town, advertise as doing handy jobs, and make a few bucks.

2. You keep going until your funds drop below a certain limit. At that point, you pull into a semi-permanent camp park and get a job in town for a few months. You continue to live in your van, but you show up at the worksite, put in your hours, and let the income accumulate until you reach a comfortable spot where you can pick up and start driving again.

3. You keep your current job and work from the road. Many corporate-type jobs are allowing employees to telecommute from home or other alternative work environments. Your employer might require you to be signed on or otherwise reachable by phone and email during certain times of certain days, so you'll

need to plan wisely to have a reliable WiFi and phone signal during those times.
4. Freelancing is another career path that is gaining in popularity. Again, you'll need a fairly continuous WiFi signal and phone connection, but if you have a talent, you might check popular contracting sites for jobs you can accomplish anywhere you choose to be.
5. The Internet. We live in an age where you can get paid for talking about yourself on the internet. If you're a talented writer, photographer, videographer, or have the gift of gab, you can consider blogging, a YouTube channel, or a podcast. You'll have the ability to charge for ad space and make money by posting sponsored ads.

There are, of course, other types of income opportunities, but the main purpose of these examples is to help you appreciate that you don't have to be a trust fund baby or have millions in the bank before you hit the road.

Depending on the lifestyle you hope to lead, the compromises you're willing to make, and the skills you're willing to learn, anyone can hit the road at any time. It's just a matter of making sure you're very prepared for all of the possibilities and realities.

Advice from the Road: Part 5

I actually started my freelancing career from the road. Because I didn't want to spend the time and effort of sending all of my friends and family postcards, I started a blog. As I was blogging, my friends would read about my adventures and share the link with their friends, and so on.

After a while, I started getting contacted by people who liked my writing style. They would have little writing projects they needed help with, and would I mind helping them out for a few bucks? Soon, I was devoting about an hour a day to these road projects.

I didn't plan to make money while on the road, but WiFi, Google Docs, PayPal, and the like make it super easy to gain a few bucks here and there. It wasn't long before I realized this was a real passion of mine, too!

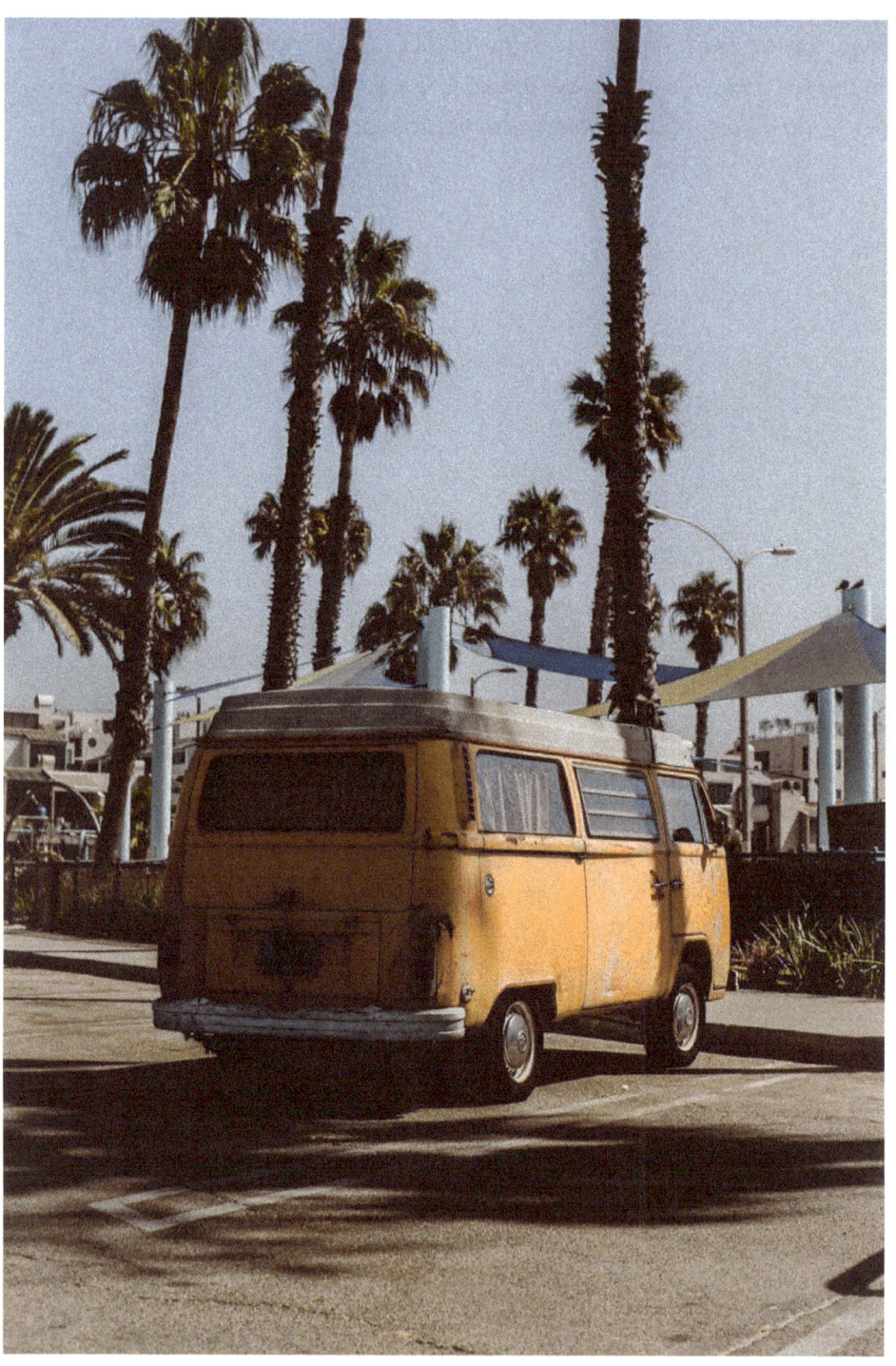

Section 4: Preparing for Your Trip

We've discussed some of the preparations in earlier sections, but this one is designed to help you get really road ready. From this section you'll be able to not only make a checklist of things to pack but have places to pack them, and an orderly system for loading and unloading everything you've got. Furthermore, when things go sideways, you'll be prepared with alternatives!

Chapter 1: Your Utilities

When you were building or buying your van or skoolie, you made some very important decisions about things like power, water, toilets, showers, and more. Here is where you make sure you're ready to hit the road with all of these things!

For your power supply, both generators and solar power have special considerations. Do you have all of the knowledge and necessities to keep your generator in good, functioning order? What is your plan for running your generator? What happens if your generator goes out? You should always have a backup plan, such as flashlights and meals that don't require heating (or a heating source that doesn't require power). Does your toilet run off the generator? That's another possibility you'll need to consider.

Where are you going to get your water? Where are you going to dispose of your greywater? What if you run out of water? What are you going to store your water in? What happens if that storage tank gets damaged?

Much like you probably have a plan at home for what to do if the power goes out or a sewer main breaks, you'll need similar alternatives when you're on the road. At the same time, your storage space will be at a premium, so whatever you choose must be as simple as possible. If you are traveling with a family, for example, perhaps the path of least resistance is checking into a hotel for the night while you repair and re-sort all of the equipment that needs attention. If you're on your own, perhaps you stay put for the night, pitch a tent, and make the most of the situation.

Chapter 2: Sleeping Arrangements

When you were building your van or buying your van, you designated space for sleeping. Now that you've built your nest, it's time to feather it!

Your bed is actually a very important part of the van life experience. After all, if you sleep poorly, you might experience unnecessary back and neck pain, or become tired more easily, or just feel generally foggy and groggy. None of these are helpful when you are supposed to be driving or having adventures.

At the same time, it's generally not practical to have a king-sized thermal adjustable massaging bed installed in your van! Thankfully, there are plenty of options on the market when it comes to creating a sleeping environment that will be comfortable for you.

Start with a solid, flat, even base. Then add a mattress layer. Because you're working in a van, you might not be able to just wander into a mattress store and grab a standard commercial mattress. Instead, you might have to do some tailoring.

Futon mattresses tend to be a great medium for the base of your mattress layer. They're designed to be rolled up or folded, so if you need to stash your bedding while you drive, a futon mattress will not be offended. They're also typically stuffed with foam or padding. This means that if you cut into one to make it the right size, you can always just adjust the dimensions of the stuffing and sew it back up. Yes, this will require a little sewing skill, but it doesn't necessarily have to be gorgeous — just rugged and functional.

One thing to keep in mind with this type of mattress is that it isn't necessarily intended to be slept on every night for long periods of time. Do your research as you shop to find one that will be durable, and take care to flip and rotate your mattress often to ensure it wears evenly.

Another option is an inflatable mattress. If you need to use your sleeping area for other functions during the day, an inflatable mattress can be deflated and stashed in a relatively small area. The only downsides to this is that you will need to re-inflate it every time you use it, and it is possible for an air mattress to get tiny rips and holes that will need to be repaired in order for you to continue using it. Furthermore, you'll need to make sure the mattress fits within the dimensions of your sleeping area. Still, there are some very sturdy and comfortable air mattresses available.

On top of the mattress layer, you can add a variety of orthopedic and temperature regulating pads, which are available at most department stores and discount stores. A simple "egg-crate"-style pad might do the job, or you might want to find something that's more sturdy, firm, and will balance out your mattress. Make sure the padding you choose can be sized to your mattress, and if you're going to roll it up and store it when it's not in use, make sure it doesn't create too much unnecessary bulk. Some of the padding on the market might be as thick (or thicker!) than your mattress which could cause storage issues.

You might also consider getting what is affectionately termed a "bug bag" if you choose a non-inflatable mattress, especially if you plan to spend a lot of time in the true wilderness. This is a waterproof, insect-proof, crumb-proof mattress cover, which typically zips to keep the mattress truly protected from all of the elements. This might seem like an unnecessary extravagance until you knock over your water bottle onto your bed in the dark or find a swarm of ants casually enjoying a crumb of food you didn't realize you dropped. If you tailor your mattress to fit the space, it might not be a perfect fit, so buy a size bigger than whatever your mattress started as. You can always use bands or clips to keep it from rustling around as you sleep. Additionally, you'll be able to store your rolled-up mattress and pad in this if necessary.

Next comes the bed sheets and linens. Go with what makes you comfortable, but doesn't require a ridiculous amount of storage. You might see glorious social media pictures of van beds stacked with throw pillows. If you need throw pillows to be physically or mentally comfortable — get them. For the most part, however, you'll need enough pillows to keep your body comfortable, a fitted sheet to keep everything together, and some assortment of blankets for your preferred sleeping temperature.

Keep in mind that temperature can be a hard thing to regulate in a van, especially if you will not have a power source. You may choose to use your sleeping bag in colder climates, or if you're going to be in hotter locations, a light sheet or nothing at all. If you enjoy sleeping with a comforter in a climate-controlled house with a fan blasting directly at you, your sleeping situation might change once you're on the road.

This is another scenario where doing a test run in your garage, basement, or corner of a room will be a good idea. Set up your mattress, pad, and all the accessories you'd like to try. See how it feels, and adjust as necessary. This way, when you finally get out on the road, you'll be in a comfortable, familiar bed.

Remember also that your sheets and blankets will have to hang out in your van. Eventually, they will need to be washed and changed. You might want to have a spare set of sheets on hand and put the used sheets in with the dirty laundry. The goal is to be minimalist, but you need to be practical, as well. If you're the type of person who can wash and dry their sheets as necessary, then you'll be able to get away with just one set.

If you do choose to bring extra bedding, make sure you store it in a sealed container or bag. If you plan on going on any outdoor adventures, you will find that mud, sand, dirt, rocks, and snow will get everywhere. Make sure your clean linen stays clean until you're ready to use it by keeping it stowed away.

Another thing to consider when it comes to sleeping and bedding is windows. Yes, windows.

If you have a skoolie, you may have a lot of windows. That can be a huge advantage because you can open them at night and let the soft night air cool you while you sleep. In addition to the night air, however, you'll also let in the insects, pollen, falling leaves and seed pods, small intelligent rodents, and any looky-loos who might want to peep the interior of your home. All of these are incredibly irritating.

For windows that you'd like to keep open, you'll want to consider screens. You might have to make these yourself. Buy the kits for this at hardware stores. The best part is they don't take much work. You'll have to decide if you want to permanently install the screens or fashion them so they can be popped in when the windows are open. The second option is going to be most convenient, but less secure. A particularly clever rodent or curious person could figure out how to pop them right back out.

What about privacy windows? If you're living in a van, it's highly likely that you have a large rear window. Tinting it for privacy is possible, but be warned that different states have different laws on how dark windows can be. Instead, you might wish to fashion a privacy curtain that can be pulled across the window at night. You can install an actual curtain or use Velcro strips adhered around the van window to hang a blanket or other fabric across the window.

When thinking about window covering, remember that anything you have in the van will get dusty and dirty (maybe even smelly!). The insides of your windows will also gather condensation from your breath as you sleep on cool nights, so make sure your window treatments aren't going to be spoiled by getting slightly damp.

Your main goals for creating your sleep setting will be comfort, climate, the ability to stow and set up quickly and easily, cleanliness, and a sense of privacy. Together, these elements can't necessarily guarantee you a perfect night of sleep, but they'll certainly help!

Advice from the Road: Part 6

The first night in our van, I imagined that everyone was looking in on me. I tried to hide with the blankets over my head, but it was so hot. Eventually, I started feeling more and more comfortable with leaving the windows cracked, and then fully open.

That's when the mosquitos came out. Great big, blood-sucking mosquitos. The van was absolutely filled with them, buzzing all night, feasting on our faces. Even in the mountains, where there was snow, they still came to visit.

We quickly put up makeshift screens in the windows, but it wasn't long before the bugs found all the holes. Our next investment was perfectly-sized screens, which we affixed to the window frame with large, industrial-strength Velcro strips. The screens stowed neatly behind the driver's seat, and extra Velcro is an easy investment.

The result was a quiet night of sleep with peaceful mountain breezes and no bug attacks!

Chapter 3: Storage Solutions

Much like power sources, storage solutions are something we've touched on several times already. As you prepare to hit the road, it's crucial to really get everything organized and accounted for.

As you pack, you'll find that there might be a few things that you don't quite have a spot for. This happens to every single person as they pack up for their maiden voyage. It is highly likely that you will overpack due to "The Unknown," which will leave you scrambling for space.

Many of us pack like we're fleeing quickly, but the good news about gearing up for your new life in a van is that you have time to be strategic and plan what you pack.

Clothing

When it comes to clothing, you're probably thinking you'll need a few daytime outfits, something comfortable to wear while driving, stuff to hike and do other outdoor activities in, and probably something civilized to wear if you decide to go out to a restaurant, museum, or other "citified" location.

It's important to note, that most clothing can do a lot of work in between washings. The jeans you wear while driving might be perfectly fine for touring a local art museum. The leggings you wear while hiking through a National Park might do the trick for driving long distances the next day.

That's not to say that clothing won't get soiled or damaged and need immediate laundry or replacement, but it's unlikely that you'll need to prepare with four pairs of pants per day. Instead, plan to hand wash anything that needs immediate attention (which you can handle in your dish tub — making the most out of everything!).

If you plan to do a lot of outdoor activities, you will want to make sure you pack plenty of clean, appropriate socks and the correct footwear. You might find yourself packing more pairs of shoes than pairs of jeans, depending on what your trip has in store for you. Hiking, running, canoeing, rock climbing or caving, and water sports all require different types of footwear, as well as storage options that can contain mud, dirt, water, and odor.

Additionally, you'll need to make sure you've got climate-related gear. Fleece jackets, water-proof windbreakers, swimsuits, and even sweaters or sweatshirts might be a great thing to pack. Just remember — you don't need to bring ALL of them.

If you're the type to overpack for a vacation, start by pulling everything you want to take with you out of the drawers and closets. Then reduce that by half. Then reduce by half again. Keep paring down until you have about seven to ten days of clothing options. You might want to check out the Capsule Wardrobe method and apply this to your overall wardrobe selection. Your goal is to carry less but to have more options.

You can always wash your clothes. You can always buy something on the road if a particular need arises. But once you're on the road, the only way to get rid of things you want to keep is to pack them up and ship them to someone who will store them for you!

Supplies

And then you've got all of your supplies. This can range from your breakdown kit to your pots and pans, to your toiletries, and so on.

If you've got built-in cabinetry, that's going to solve a lot of problems. At the same time, remember that your van or skoolie is going to be in motion. That means braking, accelerating, hard turns, winding roads, bumps, and potholes. The objects in your cabinets will shift and move, which can make a mess, or leave a bump on your head in the case of overhead bins.

Many van dwellers like to create storage solutions that prevent things from moving around too much while the van is in motion. One way to do this is to group items in plastic bins. Bins with lids can be especially helpful when it comes to making sure vital supplies don't escape and roll around while you're driving. There are also rack-style shelving solutions that can be installed in cabinets that help keep things stable. Velcro, magnets, bungee-style cords, tie-downs, and more are all very helpful resources in keeping things in place during transit, too.

If you do use bins, it's a good idea to keep them all labeled or color-coded for easy access. Additionally, make sure certain items can be accessed inside or outside the van. It's unlikely that you'll want to open the rear door and stand in the pouring rain to find a can opener.

Anything you can do to make the contents of your van stable and accessible will go a long way toward extending the comfort and usability of your van's contents. For the most part, this will take practice. Things that seem to make sense before you hit the road might take a different shape once you get used to the overall flow of van living.

Chapter 4: Emergency Kit

When you think of an "Emergency Kit," the first thing that probably comes to mind is a first aid kit. A first aid kit is an absolute necessity, but the emergency kit includes so much more. After all, you're preparing for unplanned events in a home that's on wheels, powered by many moving mechanical parts.

When thinking about what to put in your emergency kit, first consider the relatively common incidents that might occur to a motor vehicle. For example, flat tires. If you're driving a large transit bus, you're not going to be able to just head over to the shoulder and pop the spare on. But for smaller vans, a spare tire, jack, and tire iron are a great idea. You might even bring a tire patch kit, in the event of minor issues that can be addressed shortly at a tire shop.

What about jumper cables or a battery jump kit? Many of the older vans don't include automatic headlights or even an annoying buzz or beep to let you know you've left your lights on. You don't want to be stuck in the middle of actual nowhere, with no cell phone signal and no battery power.

A fire extinguisher is a very important addition to any emergency kit. Depending on the size of your vehicle, you might want to bring a few along, for the inside of the vehicle and for the vehicle itself. While a fire is unlikely, it is possible. And if you're planning to brave the wilderness? You might not be within easy access of emergency services.

A tarp may seem unnecessary. After all, vans and buses have roofs, and they're pretty leak proof. The issue is the windows. Glass is prone to cracks and breakage, and having water streaming through the inside of your van is no one's idea of a good time. While a tarp and duct tape aren't a permanent fix, they will help take care of the issue while you create a plan. Tarps also make a pretty handy landing pad, tent base, canopy for lounging outside, "spare room," and more. If you're using an outdoor hanging shower, you can use the tarp as your "floor" so you don't have to stand in mud. The uses go on and on, making a pretty convincing argument for having a tarp on hand... just in case!

Battery-operated lighting is also a good idea. This can take the form of flashlights, small lanterns, and more. Don't rely on your cell phone flashlight as a light source. If you find yourself without power and need light for a lengthy period of time, using your phone flashlight will just drain the battery. Instead, save that battery, and use a device that doesn't have the ability to call for help! Make sure you pack spare batteries as well — don't assume that you'll be able to get more whenever you need them. Batteries take up very little room and are worth it to not find yourself in a dark and scary situation.

Solar flashlights and lanterns are also fine options — just make sure you let them see the sun during the day, so they're charged when you need them.

Depending on where you're going to spend your time, you might want an emergency water purification kit on hand. While you'll largely be able to plan ahead to manage your water supply, you might find yourself in a dry location with a leak. Being able to instantly replenish your water supply is a huge benefit, no matter where you are, or what type of adventure you're having. If you're relying on a fixed freshwater tank, make sure you have a backup plan. That can even mean having a few gallons of drinking water from the grocery store on hand — just make sure you've got them stashed away in a safe location, where they can't move around and possibly spring a leak while you're driving!

Having a spare gasoline can onboard can also be helpful, especially if you're going to be traveling through long stretches of uninhabited territory. The most important consideration for having gasoline onboard is storing it properly, so it doesn't tip and spill, become too hot or too cold, or accidentally release harmful fumes into the cabin. If you have children or pets with you, you'll want to be absolutely certain they can't accidentally come in contact with the gasoline directly, either.

If you've learned some of the basics of vehicle maintenance, you'll want to have a toolset onboard also. Generally speaking, this will include a hammer or mallet, and the right-sized wrenches for all of the pieces and parts within your vehicle. You might also want a screwdriver that fits the interior screws, just in case something works loose. First-time van dwellers are always a bit surprised at what things work loose when traveling consistently over bumpy roads! There's no need to take any tools that have no use in your vehicle, so make sure you pack wisely and organize well. A small toolbox or carrying case will save you tons of frustration when you're already upset about a breakdown.

Other helpful things to have onboard are items that have plenty of practical uses. Duct tape is almost always helpful for one reason or another. From temporarily taping the soles back onto your shoes, to holding a loose cabinet door down until you can fix it, to waterproofing a baseball cap, nearly every van dweller has some zany story involving duct tape coming to the rescue in a pinch. Make sure you invest in the truly waterproof, truly sticky stuff, too.

Multi-tools, such as Leatherman or Swiss Army Knives, will prove useful in a variety of situations, as well. You'll be thrilled to have one of these in your kit when you lose the nail clippers, need to cut something to size, try to open a bottle... the list goes on and on. A pocket-sized utensil with nearly infinite uses is always welcome in a van.

Matches or a long grill-style lighter can also be helpful. If you have a propane stove or burner that you'll be using, these will be a necessity, as well as if you plan on regularly building campfires. Even if you don't plan on needing to start a fire, you might find yourself in need of a heat and light resource if you lose your power source. Camping matches are a small easy-to-store investment that could really come in handy in a pinch.

In some cases, you'll want to pack several of these items. If, for example, you're a whole family on the road, you'll probably want several flashlights, which means stocking up on more batteries. If you're going to be gone for a significant amount of time, it can't hurt to have two rolls of duct tape — one in the cabin, and one on reserve with the vehicle maintenance equipment.

Now the tricky part — where do you put all of this stuff? With the exception of items that need special storage considerations, like gasoline and water, you might choose to put everything together in a tote or cabinet that is exclusively designated for your emergency kit. However, you might want to keep some of the smaller items in an easy-to-reach spot, like the glove box, or a small in-cabin kit that can be accessed quickly. After all, it makes no sense to have a flashlight if you have to fumble around in the dark in order to find it.

When it comes to emergency supplies, there's a fine line between "too prepared" and "possible catastrophe." Just like in a stationary home, it's impossible to prepare for every eventuality. It may seem even more challenging to think of all the dangers that might befall you on the road. In order to give yourself more peace of mind, do some research beforehand on the areas where you'll be traveling. What types of perils have other van dwellers encountered? Do other travelers have recommendations for supplies to have on hand? Knowing what others have experienced in that area can help give you some perspective on your own needs so you can plan ahead.

Chapter 5: Food

The topic of food has come up several times, and for good reason — we literally cannot live without it. In our stationary worlds, we pop into the grocery store whenever we need to and load up on fresh produce, meats, cheese, eggs, frozen foods, and so on. We bring them home, organize them in our full-sized refrigerators, freezers, and cabinets, and plan to use them before the expiration date. Sometimes we don't feel like cooking, so we head out to a restaurant or order delivery, and if we order too much food, we throw that in the refrigerator and reheat it in our microwaves the next day.

It is technically still possible to do all of that in a van or bus, as long as you've got the space, power, and equipment to do so. You may not have full-sized appliances and cabinets, but you can incorporate smaller, camper-style units that do the same job. This is a very good idea if you'll be traveling with children, or if you're making van living your permanent lifestyle.

For many Van Lifers, though, there is neither room nor practical need for appliances. In reality, none of the traditional kitchen appliances are required to live. An economical use of food products, a cold storage option, and the ability to heat food and water are really all it takes to keep yourself fed on the road.

As mentioned earlier, coolers are very helpful. The type of cooler you choose does have some bearing on your food options and usage, however, An ice-chest type cooler is typically very inexpensive, and melted ice can be recycled as bathwater or used for cleaning up certain non-food items (like the floor of the van, your muddy flip-flops, etc.). The downside to this is that your cooler will fill with water as the ice melts. Unless it is replenished regularly, that means that anything in the cooler can get water-logged, and anything that gets too warm has a chance of spoiling. But, if you practice extreme discipline in the use of your ice chest, there's no reason why this can't work.

Plug-in coolers can be very helpful, too. They are generally more expensive than ice chests, but you have the luxury of never worrying about the ice/water ratio. At the same time, you've got to have the power supply to keep it going. Most units require 12 volts of power, which isn't unreasonable. If you've got an older van with no power supply, however, you might be wary of leaving it plugged in overnight, as it might drain the battery. Some coolers will have the ability to keep their contents cooled if unplugged for short periods, and some will not. Food poisoning while on the road is even more uncomfortable than it is in a house or apartment, so don't tempt the fates when it comes to food safety. Make sure your food is stored at the appropriate temperature — if your cooler can't handle it, don't take the risk.

When it comes to storing produce, you have two main goals. The first is to not have it rolling around the cabin as you drive, and the second is to not attract insects or other wildlife that might be interested in sampling your meals. Generally speaking, the cooler is a fine place to keep your fruits and veggies, even if you wouldn't technically put a particular item there at home.

As for dry foods, the goals are the same as produce, only you won't necessarily want to stash everything in the cooler. Food-safe plastic storage tubs are a very good idea for things like rice and noodles and grains, as they keep the bugs out and all of the food in one place. Canned goods and other self-storing foods(like ramen noodle packets) only need to be stored in a way that they're secure and not rolling underfoot while you're trying to drive.

Snack foods and bread products are a different consideration on the road. At home, you might roll up the bag inside the cracker box, throw a chip-clip on a bag of crispy snacks, and just keep the bread shut with a twist-tie. On the road, you've got a greater exposure to insects, and living in an open-air type environment means things will go stale and grow mold more quickly. You've also got to consider curious wildlife, as well. Make sure you can tuck your snacks and bread products somewhere safe where they won't be shared without your permission.

If you're an avid camper or outdoor fan, you probably associate foods like peanut butter, trail mix, power bars, tuna, canned stew, and ramen with living outdoors. These are certainly staples of Van Life, as well, but you can diversify your diet. The key is making sure you use everything immediately, unless you have sufficient, reliable cold storage for leftovers.

When you go to the grocery store now, you might take advantage of sales, like 3 for $10 salad kits or "fill the freezer" meat deals. Without a ton of cold storage space, that's no longer going to make sense. Instead, you'll want to purchase only what you can eat or adequately store right now.

That's not to say you can't have salad or meat but that you'll want to look at portions realistically to avoid waste.

Canned and dried food is always a go-to when it comes to living in a situation where there's not a lot of space, time, or refrigeration, but these foods are often high in sodium and preservatives. Make sure you're making wise choices for your body, health, and lifestyle. Good nutrition is key to giving you stamina and helping you maintain your health while you're on the road. Make sure you're fueling your body in a way that's appropriate for you.

When planning meals, you can always take advantage of what resources you have to create back-to-back meals that will meet the requirements of multiple food groups. For example, if you purchase one salad kit, one can of beans, a bell pepper, two tomatoes, and one large chicken breast, you can have a protein-packed chicken/bean chili for dinner with a tasty side salad, then follow it up with a big salad topped with chicken for lunch the next day. Simply cook the chicken first, then cut it into two portions — the amount you'll add to tonight's chili and the bit that you'll slice up for lunch tomorrow. Make sure you put what you're not using right away into the cooler immediately. Throw the beans, a chopped tomato, and half the bell pepper into a pot with the chicken and your favorite seasonings for a tasty "road chili." Make yourself a small salad to enjoy, too, and make sure you seal up the rest and store it in the cooler. Tomorrow, you can use the other half of the bell pepper, the second tomato, the rest of the salad kit, and the leftover chicken to have a nutritious salad.

This is just one example of how being strategic with your food and resources can help you avoid "camp food burnout." There are plenty of recipe guides for low tech and outdoor living, and we've included some links in the **resources** at the end of this book. You might feel now like having a cooler and a propane camp stove will be incredibly limiting, but the reality is that you can eat almost exactly like you do at home — you just have to scale back and be more realistic about your food use. Before you start your maiden voyage, you might want to keep track of what you cook, what you eat, how many leftovers you have, and how quickly you eat those leftovers. This will give you a little more insight about your food volume usage, so you can be more adequately prepared once you get on the road.

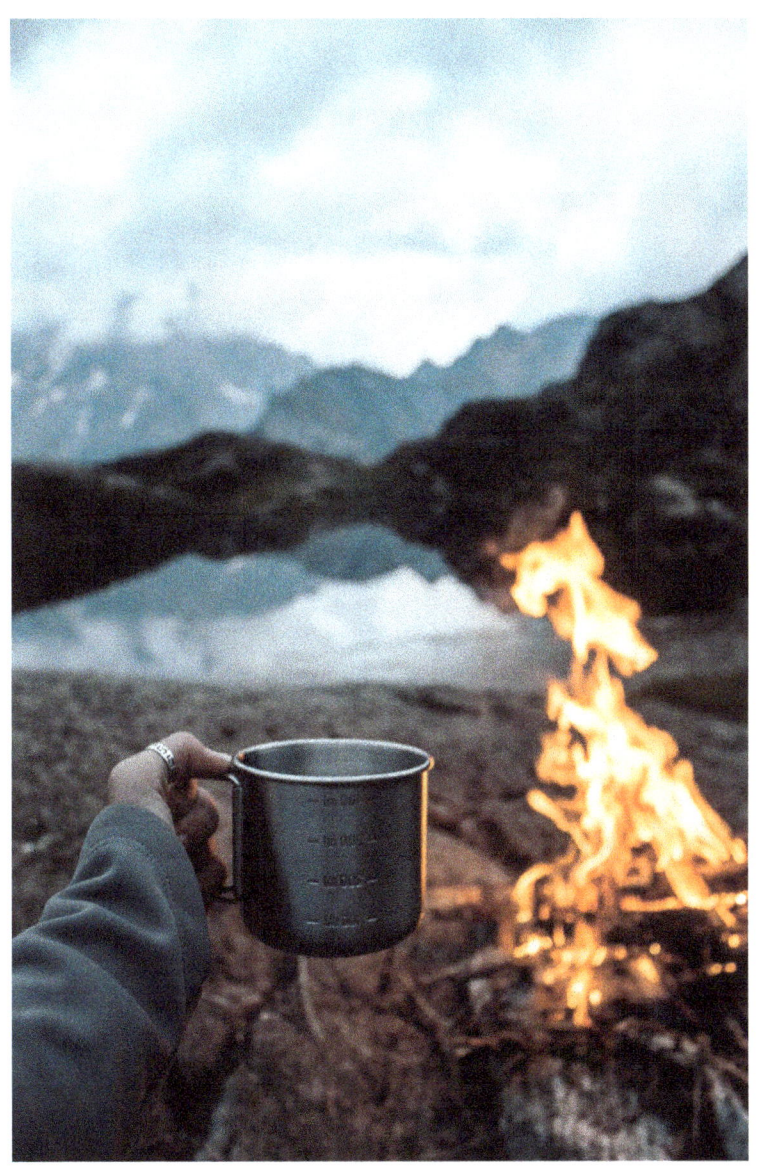

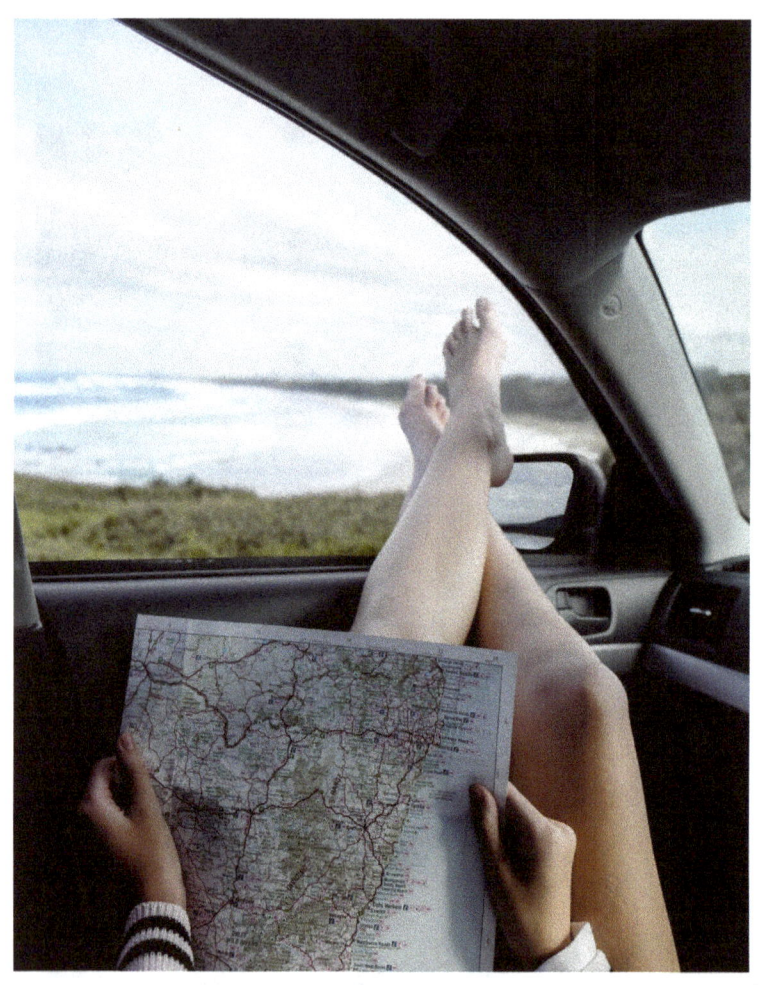

Section 5: Where Are You Going to Go?

Your van is fully packed. You're ready to go. You're equipped with all sorts of new and exciting knowledge.

So where do you go?

For some people, there's a very obvious destination in mind. Perhaps you've spent your life pining for a visit to a particular landmark, park, or museum. Naturally, you'll want to head there immediately. But the beauty of van living is that there are no destinations — only the amazing journey. Once you've hit your ideal spot — then what? You might be feeling a bit lost.

Other people might not have a clear destination selected. They might have a few general ideas of things they'd like to see, but they haven't really figured out where to go or how to get there.

Then there's a third party, which borrows a little from the first group and the second group. These folks have a definite list of things they want to see but look forward to connecting the dots with adventure.

There's plenty of grey area in between these three options, as well. If you're worried about feeling constricted by requiring plans, you'll be glad to know that there's really no wrong way to do your Van Life. It is your practice, your lifestyle, and we're just here to tap you on the shoulder and give you practical advice and suggestions. If you're the sort of person who needs guidance or help getting started, that's also not wrong. You're allowed to be confused and overwhelmed.

Let's take a look at a few different strategies that are popular among road warriors. If you're feeling too decisive, this might help you open your mind to more possibilities. If you're feeling too free, this can help you start to reach out and explore a few solid "x" marks to put on your map for future destinations.

The "Keep Moving" Strategy

Have you ever heard the phrase "goes as the wind blows?" There are van dwellers who truly do this. If they wake up and feel like checking out the west coast, so be it. Maybe the mountains next week. How about a forest?

Having a home on wheels really does mean you can go where you want, when you want, but remember that fuel costs are a very real thing. If you have an unlimited budget, perhaps driving in perpetual circles and constantly being on the move isn't a bad thing. For those who need to be aware of every cent they spend, perhaps a little bit of planning can help temper that possible spending.

Navigation is a necessary evil, even if you just want to wander. While getting lost can be fun, it does lose its novelty when bad things happen, and you don't know where you are. It can also wind up feeling a little unnecessary and uninspiring over time.

Ultimately, the "Keep Moving" strategy can turn up some wonderful roadside surprises that you never expected to find. These lifetime experiences can never be forced, anticipated, or replaced. There is so much beauty in this world, and having the freedom to experience all the beauty you can is something many people can't even imagine.

This method does require a bit of careful compromise between wandering and respecting your budget, as well as any needs you might have for bathing, laundry, and stocking up on supplies. There needs to be a bit of conscious planning but never so much that you feel restricted.

Long-Term Living

Other people like to have the opportunity to really experience the culture of a location, even if it's just for a temporary time period.

While you might stake a claim on a particular camping spot, either within a designated camp park or out in the wilderness, that doesn't mean you can't leave and explore. As discussed earlier, some van dwellers take along a scooter or bicycle, so they can leave the confines of the van to wander — you're only limited by how far you're willing to stray from the van in one day.

Much like wandering, there are both pros and cons to this type of adventure. You might end up spending more in camping fees, due to your long-term stay, but you'll likely save on your fuel budget. Even if you do your local exploration in your van, it's likely that you'll be staying within a 20-mile radius.

Additionally, you'll be familiar with the area and some of the local options. You'll establish a place to purchase groceries, do your laundry, and replenish supplies. You might find some local entertainment options that you'd never expect to experience. Locals are a great source of knowledge, input, and recommendations that you won't find anywhere else, so it might be worth it to hang out at the local watering hole and find out when the county fair is or what local band is playing soon.

At the same time, you might find yourself feeling just a little too cozy. You might start to think that you've given up one home and just moved somewhere else. Always remember — you have the freedom to start the engine and throw it into gear anytime you want. Just figure out the next place to go, and get those actual wheels in motion!

Connecting the Dots
One fun method of travel is to turn the whole experience into a wild game of "connect the dots." You can pick a handful of things you'd really like to do while you're on the road, then mosey from point to point.

There are no restrictions on this method. You choose your timeframe and how you get from Point A to Point B. The only limits that exist are those that you create. For example, if you want to go to a concert in a specific city on a specific day, you'll need to make sure you make appropriate travel plans. Otherwise, you have the freedom to wander, without the lack of direction. In many ways, this is the best of both worlds!

Advice from the Road: Part 7

Our trip started as a fifty-page list of things we wanted to see, categorized by state. Yes. You read that right — fifty pages. There was no possible way we were going to be able to squeeze everything in, and we knew that, but still, it seemed like a good way to start.

Our first step was to pull out a huge map of the United States, including major freeways. This map was really huge — it took up our entire dining room table.

Next, we used little dot stickers to plot out some of the places we wanted to go, state by state. We put everything on there. In some states, it looked absolutely ridiculous. In other states, it was clear that we had a concentration of interest in a specific area.

The plans started to take shape from there. We knew we had a limited timeframe for our first trip (if you can call a year "limited"), so we had to create a way to see as much as possible without being too indirect.

We made a few rules to make sure we kept with our desire to explore: First, we would limit our use of major freeways and take as many back roads as possible. Second, any time we stopped, we'd check out what was going on in a five-mile radius and see what we needed to check out before we kept moving on.

We cheated a little on both of those rules. We broke the "five-mile rule" a lot, and there were a few times when we were so tired, we decided to take the fastest route instead of the scenic route to make sure we were driving safely. Still, I have absolutely no regrets about the number of things we were able to see, do, and try, and the diversity of those experiences.

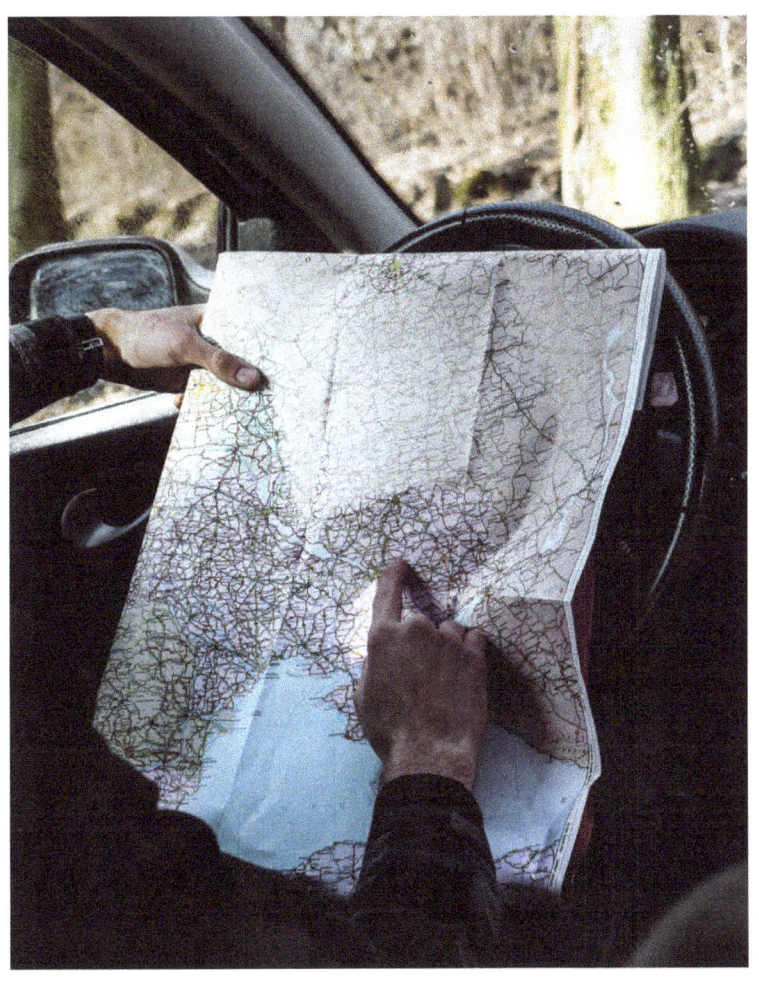

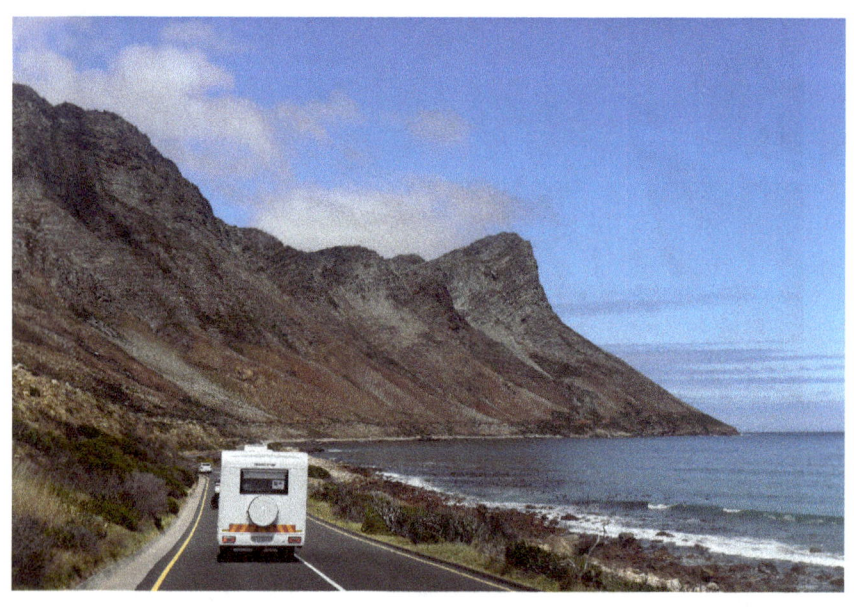

Section 6: Staying Happy on the Road

We started this book by guiding you through the Van Life mindset, to see if you're prepared for this undertaking. After all, creating an entirely new lifestyle from scratch is no small task! At this point, you've got your vehicle. It's packed. You're confidently armed with a variety of literature, including repair manuals, replacement part specs, maps, pamphlets, recipes, and so on.

You probably feel pretty well prepared for anything that could happen, and you really should feel confident with all you have accomplished up to this point. Van Life is not for the weak of heart, and preparing for life on the road is a serious rite of passage.

Still, there's really nothing that can prepare you for the feeling you'll get, sitting behind that giant steering wheel, listening to your engine complain as it climbs its first winding mountain road with you.

And there's also nothing quite like the feeling of lying awake at night, on your van mattress, wishing for the thick memory foam bed you had at home, where you can fall asleep to your favorite Netflix series without worrying about burning up the power supply, in air conditioning that you can crank when it gets hot, with a shower and a toilet that require little to no maintenance in the very next room. You might just find yourself longing for a place that doesn't kind of faintly smell like shoes and laundry all the time. That's ok! You're entirely allowed to have these feelings.

In this section, we'll focus on how to keep the motivation and feelings of well-being continue even if life is starting to feel stale. While we can't cure your melancholy, we do want you to know that this is normal and happens to absolutely everyone.

Chapter 1: Avoiding Boredom

During particularly long hauls, you will likely experience boredom. Your first reaction to recognizing this boredom may be fear. You uprooted your entire life to live on the road, only to feel the same boredom you felt at home. What is wrong with you?

The answer? Nothing. You're allowed to feel stagnant, especially when you are.

The beauty of Van Life is that you can shake it up. Celebrate that you can go anywhere. If you start feeling like "all I do is drive, and I don't even like it," then go to a National Park. Hike the trails no one hikes. Or, if you're feeling lonely, hike the trails that everyone hikes. Meet new trail buddies. Let yourself be in awe of the natural beauty that surrounds you.

If, at any time, you feel like you see the same stuff every day, you need to find some hidden gems to get you out of the rut. Hop on the internet. Go into a diner or dive bar and talk to the older locals. In your life at home, you could break out of a rut by calling your friends and doing something predictable, like meeting up for coffee or a movie or drinks. On the road, if you're feeling the monotony, you need to go meet Sue, the World's Largest Cow (or whatever is "cool and unusual" in your vicinity). Do an online search for "cool and unusual things" and a location, and you'll turn up loads of things you've never even heard about!

Find out what's going on at the local college. What bands are playing? What kind of lectures or exhibitions can you find? If nothing comes to mind, just park at the end of a street, any street, walk until you don't want to keep going, then walk back to your van. You might wonder what that will accomplish. Well, what are five things you saw during your walk that were interesting?

Keep yourself in the mindset that you have control over your exploration. Though not every place you wander will feature jaw-dropping scenery, activities that make your heart race, or experiences that open your soul, there will be plenty of things that will be new to you. Embrace these.

You'll also want to keep your mind engaged while you're on the road, with activities you can enjoy within the confines of the van. There will be bad weather days. You will probably get sick or injured. Or, you just might not feel like leaving the van on a particular day. Make sure you have plenty of stuff that will keep you engaged and entertained.

A few examples include:

- Audiobooks, music, and podcasts. You don't have to stop learning and growing, just because you're no longer a part of a wall-to-wall, brick-and-mortar society! Use this opportunity to expand your horizons. Choose audiobooks that teach you about totally new topics. Listen to performers you've only heard about from your friends. Check out podcasts that will challenge your thoughts and endear you to the human experience.
- Activity books. This may seem like it's geared to kids, but adults can gain a lot from coloring, doing logic puzzles, crosswords, sudoku, or even by trying to find Waldo! When you stare at the road for hours at a time, your mind craves something different, so put your creativity and problem-solving skills to the test with some harmless activities that won't require a lot of space or supplies.
- Blogging. Though a brief glimpse through the **resources section** may make it sound like the internet is already saturated with Van Life blogs, there's always room for your experience. You can start a blog for free and use it to share your pictures and thoughts with friends and family. You might also start a variety of social media platforms specifically for your voyage. If sharing these thoughts with the whole world isn't your style, old fashioned pen-and-paper journals are always an option.

Lastly, try to take a deep breath and remember to enjoy the moment. It is very easy for depression and anxiety to creep up on you when you're on the road, especially if you're alone. As you drive, you have lots of time to stop and reflect on negative thoughts. It's easier said than done, but don't let your mind trick you like that.

Come up with a mantra that reaffirms your abilities. You have made it this far. You have created a new lifestyle for yourself. You are doing just fine. Today is always an adventure, and you have opportunities on the road that many people will never take advantage of. Remind yourself to love what you're doing. Cherish every detail, every new experience, every little thing you've never seen before.

This is your dream, and you are making it come true.

Chapter 2: Homesickness/Loneliness

Being on the road can feel very lonely sometimes. Most of us are used to living a more sedentary lifestyle or one where we can just pick up the phone and text or call our friends. You and your buddies probably get together now and then to catch up, have dinner, watch movies, and just generally hang out. It's different when you're on the road.

You can still have friends over to your van, of course, but now you have to meet new people. You'll probably visit friends and family that you don't usually get to see while you're traveling, but all the people you see every day will be exactly where you left them.

While this concept might make you feel very sad, that's not entirely bad news. They're exactly where you left them. You can go visit them. Some people feel that, since they're devoted to Van Life now, they can't go home. It's ok to go home.

There is going to come a time when both your body and soul will long for the comforts and conveniences of home. If you have the desire to go back to the place where you started your journey, go for it! Stay with friends or family back in your hometown. Go to your regular haunts. Everyone will want to hear stories, so share them! Soon, your heart will long for the road again, and off you'll go, spiritually refreshed from your visit.

You might also try planting for a bit wherever you are on the road. Find a long-term parking solution, and let yourself have a routine for a few days. Sometimes the brain and body need a sense of regularity and stability to help you put everything into perspective.

Additionally, keep your finger on the pulse of the van community. There are plenty of meetups scheduled throughout the year, even around the world. You might start conversing with your new best friends via the forums, blogs, and social media sites dedicated to those living the Van Life. Becoming a part of a community can help you with those feelings of longing and belonging.

Advice from the Road: Part 8
The first time you miss an important family event, it will break your heart. You'll see the pictures online — maybe your whole family enjoying cake together — and you'll wish you were there. You'll be able to feel all the hugs, hear the laughter, smell the over-cooked casserole, and your heart will cry out.

The first event I missed was my niece's birthday party. It was a small shindig, and really not a big deal, but when I saw the pictures of her opening her gifts, beaming at the camera, surrounded by torn wrapping paper and the bounty of her party, I cried. I wanted to be there. But it wasn't practical to be there and here, 800 miles away in the middle of the mountains.

Sometimes, you'll feel like you've done something selfish. People will try to tell you that, too. But the reality is that we all choose the lifestyle that's best for us.

You can choose to come home for the holidays, the birthdays, the anniversaries, the bachelorette parties, and so on. But the realities of time and space mean that you can't be in two places at once. You can't summit Angel's Landing and be in Florida by dinner time.

Remember that you can make room for everything and anything that you value, but you don't have to make room for everything and anything that's suggested to you. You can always go back. You can always come back. Don't let yourself feel rushed or pushed.

One tool that I began to value from the road was phone calls. It's so easy to get away with texting conversations, but when you're on the road, hearing someone's voice can be very soothing. It's also likely that there's someone who wants to hear from you, too. When you have a fully-charged battery and service, reach out — make a call. Talk. It'll do your soul some good.

Chapter 3: Housekeeping

Housekeeping might not be the most enjoyable use of time, but it's extremely necessary. If you're the type who has a "junk drawer," a "mail folder," or "a laundry chair". You might find Van Life challenging at first.

In a van, any mess you make is proportionately larger than it would be in a house or apartment. If you leave a pair of shoes on the floor of your bedroom, you can probably maneuver around them pretty easily. If you leave your shoes on the floor of your van, you will trip over them, and you will get mad at yourself for leaving them where you could trip over them.

Living in close quarters requires a new level of hygiene, which can be especially tricky when you don't have the ability to give yourself hour-long exfoliating showers every day. Keeping the stinky things stored, as we mentioned earlier, is a great way to prevent a long-term, permanent reek, but you'll still need to wash everything regularly. That includes yourself, your laundry, your bed linens, any rugs you might have, your dishes, and your commode, just to name a few. Make sure you dispose of spoiled food immediately. If you are practicing recycling on the road, make sure your empties are rinsed.

Not only do these practices cut down on bad smells, but they also cut down on bugs and critters. Wildlife is a very real part of Van Life and can include everything from the innocuous visits of birds, squirrels, and chipmunks, to the possibly dangerous curiosity of bears. You'll definitely want to avoid the headache of an ant infestation, but there's no reason to tempt a hungry grizzly!

To avoid all of this, make sure you sweep your abode on wheels regularly. Clean up any spills immediately. Get rid of trash as frequently as you can. Do your part to keep things as clean as possible.

Not only does this practice have sanitary implications, but it can also make you feel better about your dwelling. Some people feel a sense of purpose and pride when they mow their lawn or scrub their floors in a stationary home. Doing something as simple as washing all of the mud from your latest off-road excursion can remind you that you love your new home and your new life, and you wouldn't have it any other way!

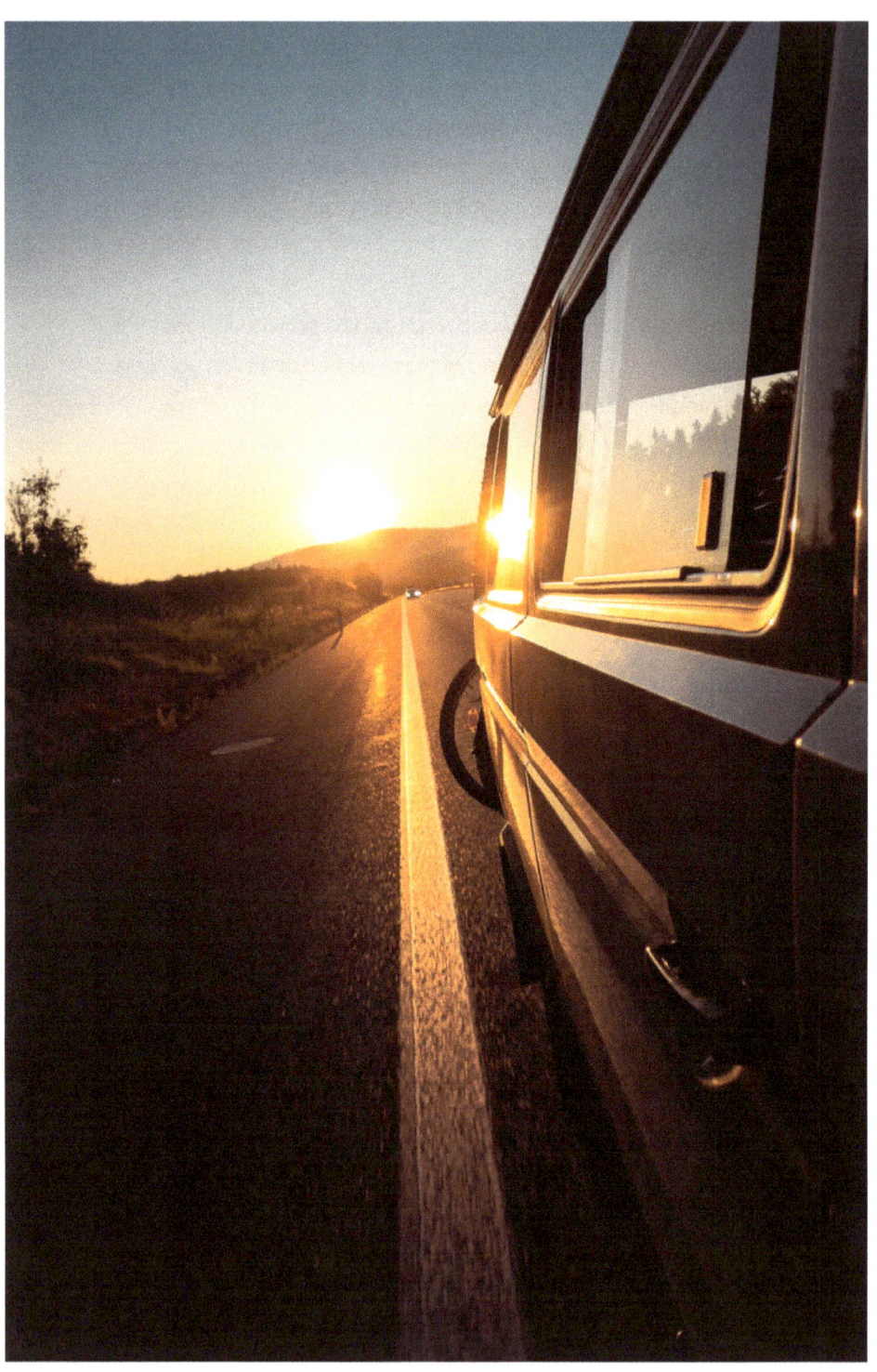

In Conclusion

Is Van Life for everyone? No. The truth is that most people won't even consider, think about, or be able to fathom the idea of living in a small, mobile space. The idea of not knowing where you're going to sleep tonight, or heating up beans over a propane burner in the dark, or going to the bathroom outside at midnight might sound like an absolute nightmare to some people.

But there is a special breed of people. There are some who hear or read phrases like this, and their hearts beat a little faster and a little harder. The ideas of "opportunities" and "unknowns" sound more welcoming than fearsome. They look at the walls around them and feel like they're being crushed by stability. These are the people who are born Van Lifers.

Are you one of them? Only you can tell for sure. If there is one thing we hope you've learned from this book, it's that you can't do Van Life the wrong way. Beyond that, building your own Van Life is a process and not one that comes quickly or easily.

Can you find "any old" van, start the engine, and take off? Sure! There are some people who are naturally adaptive. But for those of us who are taking off from what feels like a very sheltered spot, there can be lots of planning and attention to details in order to feel more secure about this huge decision.

If there's one piece of advice all van dwellers should know, it's "Don't panic when things go wrong — they just will." The first time things go topsy-turvy, it will be terrifying. There will be setbacks. You will revisit the drawing board many times. The good news is that, even when things go upside down, they tend to put themselves right sideup again, as long as you don't panic.

Remember also that this isn't a competition. Just because someone on social media does it differently, doesn't mean you've failed. If you catch a cold and spend two days in a hotel recovering, that doesn't mean you're inadequate. It means you did the best thing you could for yourself in that situation. If you choose to start the day with your favorite chain restaurant doughnut and coffee, don't feel like your experience is any less authentic than the bloggers who figure out how to make overnight oats in a tin coffee mug. Just make sure you budget for the expense and get on with your best Van Life.

In short, be sure to enjoy every step of the journey. You are doing something many people dream of, but very few people get to experience.

This is the beginning of your new life.

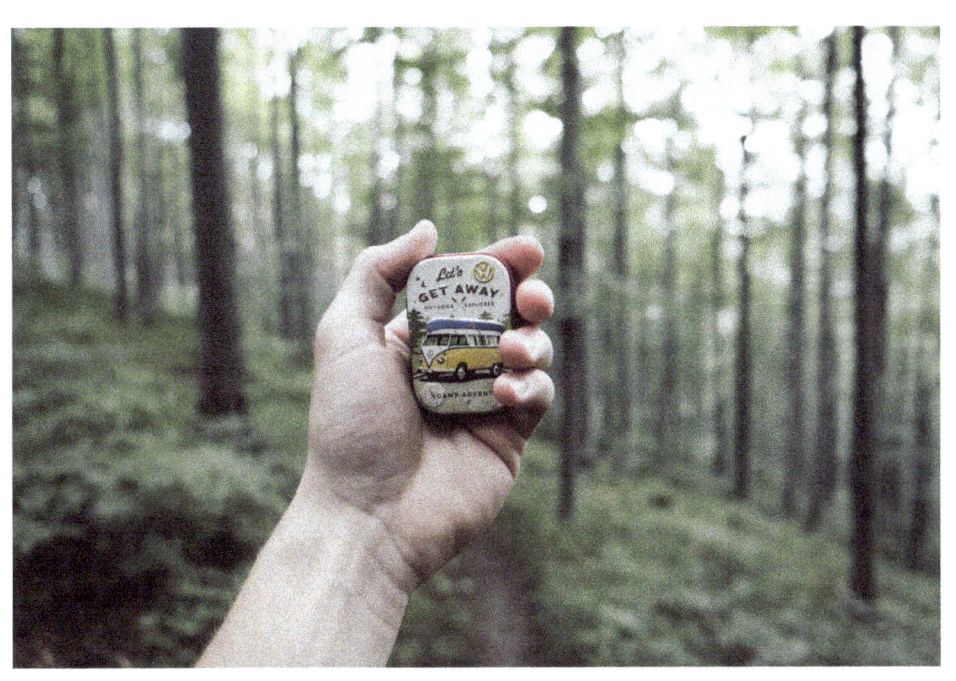

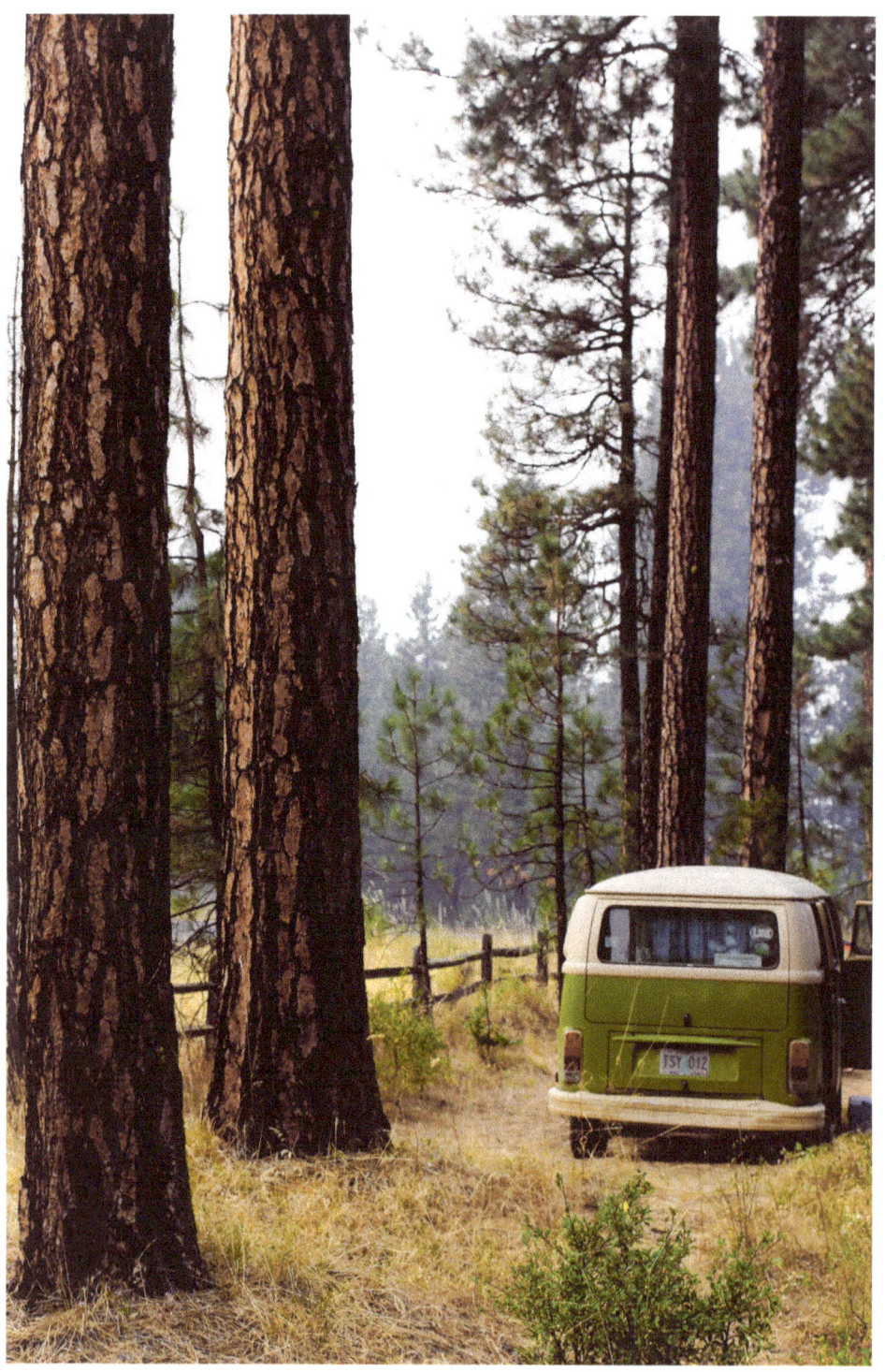

Section 7: Helpful Resources for Future Van Dwellers

The following links lead to online blogs, reference materials, and websites that can help you with every step of the process of converting to Van Life. The views and ideas expressed in each of these links belong solely to the person writing it, so please don't consider their inclusion an endorsement or partnership. We simply wanted to get you started on the quest for more information.

Remember, there is no "wrong" way to do Van Life. There are only ways that work better for your lifestyle and things that don't work for you. It's a very personal experience that often requires a lot of trial and error.

Still, sometimes it helps to read the experiences of those who have tried it, are doing it, or are in the same position as you are when it comes to trying something very, very different.

Feel free to check out some of these links to draw inspiration, and continue your quest for more information!

The Van Life State of Mind:
As noted, you've got to be in the right headspace to really enjoy the wild ride.

http://www.alwaystheroad.com/blog/2017/3/24/is-van-life-for-you-how-to-know-if-its-right-for-you

Parking Options, Camping Options, and Sleep Spots
Tracking down a spot where you can catch up on some rest or spend the night can be challenging, especially when you're on a tight budget. Here are some resources to help you find a safe, practical place to rest.

https://www.campendium.com/camping/vanlife/
http://thevanual.com/sleeping-and-safety/

https://www.cheaprvliving.com/stealth-city-parking/bobs-12-commandments-for-stealth-parking-in-the-city/
https://divineontheroad.com/overnight-parking/
https://kombilife.com/van-life-free-camping/
https://www.classicvans.com/
https://www.youtube.com/watch?v=oqPiP2JYVNc
https://www.nps.gov/index.htm

Choosing a Van

If the topic of vans as a vehicle is new to you, you'll definitely want to do additional research before starting the shopping process. Here are a few sites that will help you learn more about the types of vans and buses, as well as a variety of opinions to help guide you through the pros and cons of every option out there.

https://www.curbed.com/2018/1/31/16951486/best-van-conversion-rv-camper-vanlife
https://vanclan.co/best-van-to-live-in/
https://gnomadhome.com/why-choose-conversion-van-for-vanlife/
https://gearmoose.com/van-life-best-camper-vans/
https://weretherussos.com/van-chassis-camper-van-conversion/

Classic Van Lifers

As mentioned, Classic vans have a following of their own. Here are some links to resources for people who are living the "old school" way, with vans from earlier eras. Check out their thoughts, experiences, and words of advice.

https://bearfoottheory.com/category/van-life/
https://blog.feedspot.com/van_life_blogs/
https://vanclan.co/vanlife-blogs/

Skoolies

For those who are interested in larger format on-the-road living, buses are the way to go. The conversion, rehab, remodel, and updating of these vehicles could be a book on their own, so we've included a few links to folks who have gone through the process. Their insights, advice, trials, and tribulations can be helpful as you adjust to the learning curve of a great big diesel vehicle!

https://gearjunkie.com/school-bus-rv-camper-conversion-remodel
https://www.curbed.com/2019/3/6/18246221/camper-conversion-skoolie-vanlife-tiny-house
https://www.buslifeadventure.com/index.php/blog/16-blog/198-bus-life-vs-van-life-as-seen-through-the-eyes-of-a-van-dweller

The Cost of Van Living

While we've included some details about how to calculate your van shopping budget, your remodeling budget, your road budget, your overall experience budget and more, we can't predict all of the expenses that might go into your individual experience. Check out these resources for more inspiration.

https://www.moneyunder30.com/van-living
https://www.parkedinparadise.com/van-life-cost/
https://mymoneywizard.com/living-in-a-van/
https://www.explorist.life/how-much-does-van-life-cost/
https://faroutride.com/vanlife-actual-cost/

Generating Revenue on the Road

Again, we all need to follow our own path when it comes to careers, so only try this at home if you think you can make it work with your own skills, talents, and preferences. If you're feeling hesitant about trying to make a career work on the road, here are some thoughts, ideas, and words of wisdom from those who have made it happen.
https://www.thewaywardhome.com/make-money-living-on-the-road/

http://www.alwaystheroad.com/blog/2017/9/18/the-ultimate-van-life-question-answered-how-we-make-money-on-the-road
https://projectvanlife.com/van-life-money-tips/
https://vansage.com/remote-jobs-for-van-life/
https://outboundliving.com/working-making-money/
https://vacayvans.com/how-to-make-money-working-remotely-living-vanlife/
https://wandrlymagazine.com/article/make-money-in-a-van/

On the Topic of Food

Everyone has different tastes, so we tried to round up a bunch of links that cover food storage, food preparation, and on-the-road recipes that many people can relate to. The food suggestions we mentioned within the chapter aren't inclusive of all diets and preferences, so we wanted to help get the creative cooking ideas flowing with a handful of resources.

https://www.climbonmaps.com/cold-food-storage.html
https://authenticavl.com/van-life/how-to-keep-your-food-fresh/
https://vanclan.co/vanlife-recipes/
https://mpora.com/camping/12-super-simple-meals-for-when-youre-living-in-a-van/
https://www.vancognito.com/van-life-cooking/
https://www.allrecipes.com/article/three-ways-to-conquer-camper-van-cooking-vanlife/
https://vansage.com/easy-campsite-recipes/
https://theplaidzebra.com/these-5-cheap-and-easy-meal-ideas-will-give-you-the-freedom-to-take-life-on-the-road/
https://simplyvanlife.com/non-perishable-foods-for-van-life/
https://www.parkedinparadise.com/storage-organization/
http://www.nomadswithavan.com/van-friendly-foods/
https://www.youtube.com/watch?v=1zTzaeOo8_w

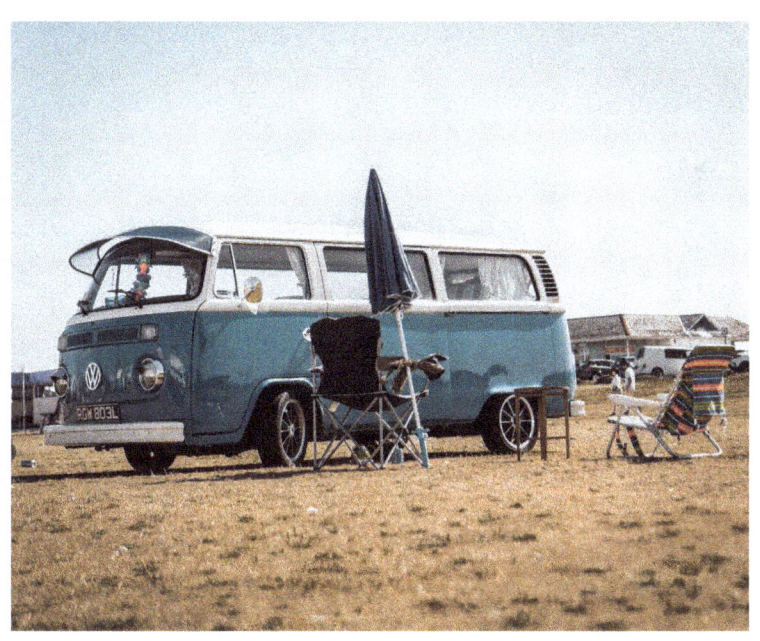

WORKING WHERE YOUR HEART IS:

FINDING SUCCESS OUTSIDE THE TRADITIONAL OFFICE

Kristine Hudson

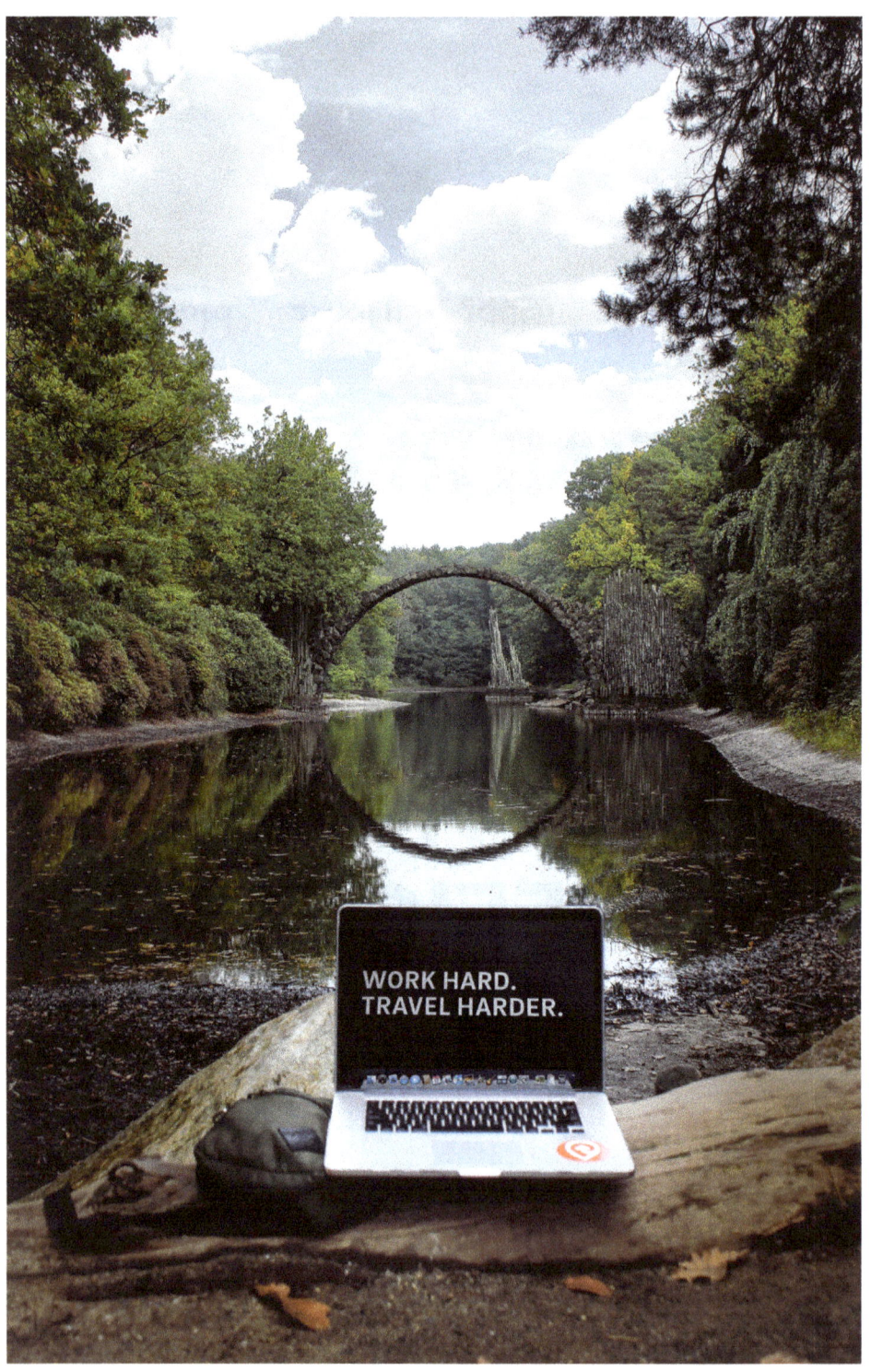

Section One: The Here and Now of Working on the Run

Introduction: Why Do I Need This Book? What Will I Learn?

Not too long ago, the concept of "working remotely" was reserved only for the lucky few. In fact, many larger corporations mistakenly believed that workers were most productive and provided the most value for the employers' investments when they were seated at a company-supplied desk, in a deliberately organized cubicle formation, with a corporate-issued phone and computer. Occasionally, a top-level executive would take his or her work on the road while attending a productivity conference half a world away. Perhaps, after a great deal of deliberation, an expecting mother would be given the access to log in while on bed rest. These situations were few and far between.

One may argue whether it was the general success of these work-from-home pioneers that paved the way for the modern trend of working remotely. Others point out that the catalyst of this movement was the resulting rebellion from those who asked "if they can do it, why can't we?" Though both parties have made valid contributions to the increasing number of people who telecommute to their jobs on a regular basis, much of the thanks can be attributed to ever-evolving technology and security protocols, which have made the notion of working from anywhere BUT a cubicle a more regular practice.

The phrase "working remotely" has evolved since the early days of being a rare privilege. While many think of it as "working from home," the truth is that technology has advanced light years in the past 30 years, which has taken the concept from just a home office, to almost anywhere as long as you can get a reliable phone signal (that can then be converted into a Wi-Fi Hotspot!).

The fact that we can work from anywhere offers endless possibilities. Not coincidentally, the number of individuals living the nomadic "van life" dream has also increased dramatically. For many people, the conclusion is obvious: the time has come to work on the road.

Now that you're considering working remotely, you're probably feeling refreshed and incredibly inspired by this imminent taste of freedom. You may feel ready to go. Just boot up your laptop, and the workday starts, right? Well, unfortunately it's not so simple.

In the following chapters, we are going to look at working remotely from the inside, out. Thanks to the early pioneers of the work from home, or "WFH" movement, today's workers can learn the intricacies, difficulties, rewards, and challenges of leaving the office behind. There are many reasons why one might choose to make this change and, whether you do so regularly or intermittently, it's a great idea to know what you're getting into before you take the leap.

Perhaps you are just starting to kick around the idea of working remotely. Maybe you're getting the sneaking suspicion that winding your way through endless traffic twice a day, only to stare at the same walls for the majority of your working hours isn't the way you want to live. Regardless of how much you love your job, a lot of your engagement level as an employee comes from the environment in which you work. If you find yourself overly stressed about your commute, your office space, your coworkers, or all of the above, your productivity will most likely decline. You may find yourself more focused on your emotional situation than the tasks you need to accomplish. At this stage, perhaps you're thinking about proposing the idea of working remotely to your manager, but you're not sure how to approach it, or if it would even be a good idea.

Or maybe that's not you at all. You may be perfectly happy working in the office. You could not be happier with your job, and you cherish the time you spend in your car, catching up on your favorite podcasts. Maybe the social aspect of your office inspires you. That being said, there may be something that frequently drags you away from the office. Maybe you have a child or family member who requires attention. It could be difficulties with your own health. You might just feel drawn to a lifestyle that involves a change of scenery. For any number of reasons, it's far more practical in your situation to step away from the office building and work where you are physically needed. You might be wondering if this is the right decision, and how you can get all your ducks in a row before you start moving things out of your cubicle.

Then again, you may have already jumped ahead to the "remote" part, and now you need to pick up on the "working" thing. It's not unusual to put the cart before the horse- or in this case, the van before the bank account. Some folks quit their jobs for a life of adventure, enjoy a span of freedom, then gradually return to the working world once their money situation becomes too tight.

There's no "one true way" to do WFH, just as there isn't a "correct" van lifestyle or one "perfect" way to do any given job. In fact, you may have absolutely no desire to live in a van or travel the roads- you just want to have the option available if that desire did arise. For some, the freedom of working remotely may be working at the very edge of the 5G service areas. Others may reflect that freedom by wearing a bathrobe and sipping iced tea on the back porch while conducting a meeting.

Your ideal setup might be working from a designated work space within your home. WFH is a great situation for many people. You might want to have the flexibility to work from anywhere, or "work remotely." Some larger companies offer an option they term "telecommuting," which gives you the advantage of never directly working with anyone- you simply call in whenever necessary and otherwise submit work via email or cloud. Many remote workers are even able to alternate between these different forms. One day might be spent at the home office, another might be spent on the road while heading to client onsite meetings, and other days might be spent tied to the telephone.

Regardless of where you want to work, the concepts of working on the run are shared amongst nearly everyone who is ready to walk away from the cube farm and into the world of earning an income from literally anywhere else. Whether you're setting up office from the back of your converted skoolie, or from your Manhattan apartment, many of the following tips will be helpful for transitioning successfully. In this book, we'll cover many common concerns, including connectivity and scheduling. We'll take a look at how to set up a workspace that helps you stay productive and inspired as well as maintaining peace of mind and reducing stress throughout the transition. You may not have considered how your life will change once you introduce work into your living situation, but you will likely experience some significant physical, mental, and psychological shifts.

Though transitioning from a static office job to work on the run is very, very rewarding for many people, it's also a decision not to be taken lightly. There are preparations to be made throughout every aspect of your life. This is especially true if you are coordinating your work transition with other life changes. While some of these may be intuitive to a seasoned office worker, many of us are not aware of what we take for granted until something goes awry. The purpose of this book is to keep you focused and mindful of those things which can be complicated, challenging, or not yet apparent.

Working on the run is not for everyone. By reading this book, you will be able to better determine whether your work style and lifestyle are conducive to working outside of the office environment, office hours, or both. After we've discussed the considerations of making the transition, we'll go over the job options best suited to a nomadic lifestyle, and strategies on conditioning your mind and environment to help you become your most productive self, no matter how distracting your surroundings may be. Working remotely requires a lot of self-discipline, but for those with the right attitude and preparation, it can be one of the best decisions of your life.

Chapter One: My Own Journey to "Working on the Run"

In retrospect, there's nothing in my upbringing that would've suggested that I would choose the type of lifestyle I've chosen. Starting from a young age, my parents made it a point to take me on exciting adventures several times a year.

Sometimes we'd journey via plane from our home in Ohio to highly exotic locations (at least, in my young and impressionable eyes), such as the seashores of Florida. We once stayed at a friend's condo, where I was completely entertained by the tiny lizards that would zip around the patios and sidewalks. This may seem super mundane for many readers, but for a preschooler from the suburbs, this was an amazing experience.

Other journeys were less exotic but still offered excitement with the added bonus of being educational. We'd visit museums in Columbus, Cleveland, and Cincinnati. We would drive down to the American South to visit family members for the holidays and watch the brisk Northern weather warm through car windows that would eventually be rolled down as the temperatures climbed. I was obsessed with horses, so we made it a point to check out the Kentucky Horse Park, and Chincoteague Island.

These trips were the high point of my boring suburban existence. As a child, I'd become thrilled with the idea of taking a two hour car trip to my cousins' house, simply because I knew I'd see new things. When I gained the freedom that comes with a driver's license and my own semi-reliable vehicle, things really took off. In college, I'd quietly creep off with a friend or two to check out any place that might be more exciting than the small town in which I lived- Chicago, Detroit, Pittsburgh.

You would think that being twenty something, postgraduate, with a brand new pile of bills to pay would have calmed down my urge to explore a bit, but I managed to land a fancy corporate job, and as my career flourished, so did my paychecks. I also came equipped with the standard responsibility level of a young college grad, which is to say I managed to keep myself and my cat alive, but the rest of my choices were somewhat questionable.

As a result, my bonuses and raises were spent on travel. I went to Boston, Baltimore, and Washington DC. My time off accrued as I put in long hours and late nights at the office, eking my way ahead in the corporate world, and I'd cheerfully fritter it all away by meeting up with friends and family all over the country.

Fast forward about ten years, and things couldn't be more different. I was still working for a large corporation, but now I had become completely disillusioned with the whole thing. My career had really taken off, but I hadn't had a vacation that hadn't been consumed with work in several years. Sure, I still travelled- in fact, I fell in love with hiking and backcountry excursions shortly after I met my husband Brad, but I also remained tied to my Blackberry in case I got an urgent client email. I even got a crisis call from a client while I was attending my grandmother's funeral. It was all too much for me.

After one weekend of backcountry and hiking, which had been unsurprisingly cut short by some payroll calculation crisis or another, I remember driving home thinking, "there's got to be another way." It's not that I hated my career, but I was angry at how much of me was devoted to answering phone calls, emails, and dealing with other people's problems, when all I wanted to do was stare off into a brand new horizon and let the amazing views, cultures, scenes and people of this planet sink into my soul.

That's when I saw it, puttering over the horizon towards us. It was old, and brown, but in pristine condition. I turned to Brad and said, "What if we dropped everything and lived in a VW bus?" Shockingly, he didn't drive off the road. I think he said something to the effect of "yeah, that would be cool." In the grand tradition of spouses everywhere, I think he was giving me about 45% of his attention.

Much to the astonishment of everyone privy to the plan, we turned the key in the ignition of our 1985 VW Vanagon about three years later. I can't say "and we never looked back," because there was a lot of second guessing, regret, fear, and tears that first year. If you've ever coasted down the highway during rush hour with a giant cloud of black, noxious smoke following you, you're probably familiar with the feeling of wanting to teleport yourself to another dimension, ASAP.

But, we stuck with it. Here we are, on the road, and while I'd love to say "since we were fabulously wealthy, we never had to work again," that would be a lie. Overall, our daily living expenses have dropped dramatically. We still enjoy eating, doing laundry, putting gas in the van, and the occasional hotel room when we find ourselves getting super grumpy about dirt, inclement weather, and especially bugs.

As with all of my books to date, what you're about to read comes from years of personal experience, including many experiments: some that failed miserably, and some that succeeded brilliantly. Both Brad and I work on the road, but we have very different types of jobs. He's still in the corporate space, sweating through twelve hour conference calls, while I'm a freelancer.

The question we field the most is whether we actually earn money? The answer is yes, of course. We're charitable people, but we do the work so we can get paid. We have bank accounts and expenses, just like everyone else. Our pay is set up as a direct deposit. Brad is paid bi-weekly, and I'm paid shortly after each deadline I meet.

This book will walk through many of the decisions and situations I and others who work from the road have had to consider along the way. While I will share my own experiences, the topics that I cover will be familiar to anyone who has made the transition from an office setting to WFH, remote worker, or telecommuter status. I've interviewed others who have gone from a traditional office setting to the view of their choice, and I have researched the advice of experts and those who have been doing this far longer than Brad and I have.

One thing to bear in mind is that every experience will be different. While Brad and I don't have children, for example, I've been sure to interview couples who are working on the road with families. In short, it would be impossible to be able to cover every "what if" scenario. Instead, I've chosen to write about some of the very common struggles, decisions, and considerations that many people have experienced when leaving the office behind to pursue the work environment of their dreams.

Next we'll take a look at why you might wish to follow in the footsteps of so many others and take your job away from the office environment. There are many minute details you'll want to consider. The goal of this book is to prepare you for those little bumps in the road before you encounter them.

Whether you're rethinking your decision to work on the run, or just starting to consider the possibilities, know that you are not alone, and that there is a practical solution for every situation that occurs!

Chapter Two: Where Are You? An Exercise in Learning More About Yourself

If you're reading this book, then working from your home or anywhere outside the office is clearly on your mind. It might be the start of an idea, or you might be fully engaged in the process. Either way, you know your intention, but the road to success might not be as obvious as you hoped it would be.

The first hurdle that has to be cleared is purely psychological: WHY do you want to work remotely?

It may not feel like it yet, but this is actually a pretty big decision to make. Many things will change by leaving the office, and whether or not those changes feel beneficial or too difficult will depend greatly on your lifestyle, your attitude, and your overall mental state.

At this stage, you'll likely have a cloud of thoughts buzzing around your mind. Organization is the key. Whether you're the type who likes to jot lists or keep a journal, or the type who requires a linear system like swimlanes or an Excel spreadsheet, it's important to keep track of these thoughts. Like insects swarming a campfire, they'll quickly retreat, only to be replaced with new concerns and details.

So let's start by creating the first list or spreadsheet to answer the questions below :

> *How did you get here?*
> *Why do you want to work remotely?*

There may be a myriad of answers to these questions, but make sure to take the time to write them all down. No one else has to read this list or sheet, so you have nothing to hide. Include everything from the most major concerns ("I feel trapped in this lifestyle") all the way down to the petty ones ("There's never coffee left by the time I get to the office and I have to buy my own"). Everything that's on your mind is valid at this point. Don't fool yourself into thinking this is a simple black-and-white situation. Explore your list and consider what having your time and location to yourself can help you accomplish in the long run.

Many people have a hard time starting this exercise. There are so many thoughts and emotions that come to mind when considering the activities that take up most of your waking hours. It might help you to walk through your daily experience so you can identify pain points or things for which you are grateful on a step-by-step basis.

While everyone's office experience is a bit different, chances are that your day in the office looks something like this:

1. You wake up every morning to choose an outfit that meets someone else's dress code.

2. You drive through mind-bending traffic to the office building someone else has selected, sitting in a chair you don't like at the desk that has been assigned to you.

3. Your coworkers are decent enough, but you spend the majority of the day in the company of people you don't know, using equipment that dozens of others have used before you. Both you and the

equipment are assigned identification numbers, rather than having an actual identity.

4. The highlight of your days is usually taking breaks at the appointed times to escape to a limited number of places that can be accessed in the allotted span of the break. Alternately, you sit at your desk, checking out only the websites that the company firewall permits you to view, or trying to get a signal on your phone so you can take a quick peek at your social media or texts.

5. If all goes well, you are permitted to leave the office at the regularly scheduled hour, but sometimes you have to stay late to finish a task, work with a customer, or deal with piles of work. If you're paid on an hourly basis, you might enjoy the overtime pay, but if you're salaried, it may not be so exciting.

6. Then you get another mind-bending commute home, in which you attempt to relax and shake off the challenges and stress of the day, have a peaceful dinner, and get some sleep before it all repeats again the next day.

As you read this list, some or all of it may resonate with you. Alternatively, there may be some sections that don't speak to your experience. Naturally, this isn't going to be reflective of every person's specific situation, but the experience described above is common amongst those who work in an office building. What types of images or feelings come up as you read through this example? Where do those thoughts and emotions belong on the list or sheet you are creating?

For example, you might be feeling restricted and stifled as you read this list. You may feel that your workplace has too many rules and regulations. Maybe you feel there are too many decisions being made for you.

You may notice that in this example, there's very little flexibility for the incidental occurrences of daily life. This type of working model expects bodies in seats for a specific amount of time each day. So if you or a family member have an appointment, you'll likely have to take at least part of the day off, especially with travel time factored in. Depending on your company's time off policies, you may or may not get paid for that time away from your desk.

Time off might be hard to come by as well. While you may yearn to spend summer days at the beach with your family, that might also be the busy season for your business, which means watching the sunset from your desk, rather than from a gorgeous oceanfront.

If there's an accident or emergency, you've got to work things out with your job before you can give full attention to the situation. While many managers are understanding, a quick google search will reveal plenty of horror stories in which an incident that could have been resolved with a little sympathy results in the loss of a job… or worse.

One major draw towards working remotely is control. When you take your job offsite, you often gain control over much of your daily work experience. That can include everything from the hours that you work, to where you work, and when and how you spend your lunch hour.

Working remotely doesn't guarantee that you'll be able to breeze through every appointment, spend every day lounging at the beach, or ensure that nothing bad will ever happen. It just means that you'll have the ability to make minor adjustments based on your real-life needs, rather than spending a strict eight hours each day writhing under the control of your boss, your coworkers, or your customers. If you need a bathroom break, you can typically take one, instead of waiting for your scheduled-and-approved morning breaktime. If you need to drop your car off for an oil change during your lunch break, your boss can not tell you that you're not allowed to leave the premises until you clock out for the day.

You may find the idea of having this level of control very appealing. Rather than having to schedule time off for an appointment, you simply schedule your meetings and calls around that appointment. You mark the time as unavailable, and you make up the time by starting work earlier or working later. And instead of having to skip out on the family vacation year after year, perhaps you head down to the beach and watch the waves roll in as you field essential calls and emails.

Is it complete freedom? No, of course not. You still need to do the job you're getting paid to do. Your boss, Human Resources department, and overall corporate entity can still dictate the rules, and you still need to be crystal clear in all communication with coworkers and customers alike. But in this situation, working remotely gives you a greater level of control, from being able to take calls in your pyjamas, to logging in from a lounge chair.

Perhaps you want to take that even further. You don't just want to work from home- you want to work for yourself. Not everyone has to go the full nine yards like I did, leaving home and work behind to live in a van like a hippie and write all day. There are, however, many opportunities for those who wish to run a side-hustle or even a full-time gig from home or from the road. Predictably, many of these gigs offer even greater opportunities for control, and allow you to have almost complete flexibility over your hours as long as you are still completing any set projects and meeting your deadlines.

So, as you're making your list, lanes, spreadsheet, or idea map, keep these concepts in mind. You may find yourself starting to group your reasons into categories, such as "Things I Need to Control," or "Areas Where I Need Flexibility."

Kristine's List

For me, having control has always been a huge part of the decisions I've made, especially within my career. My transition from college to corporate life was pretty rough. I felt like I had to prove myself every single day. It wasn't unusual for me to work shifts of twelve hours or more, day after day after day. Ultimately, I was very successful in my role and made a huge impression on people at the executive level. But none of that saved me when the division I was working for was sold. The new company didn't have my role within their organizational structure, and since no one could figure out what to do with me, I was dismissed.

I was given a very healthy severance package with a huge financial incentive to stay "on call" for the remainder of the year. I did what most people who have suddenly had the rug pulled out from under them do. I made a series of irrational decisions that mostly involved not staying at home and moping. I traveled, hiked, and camped, distracting myself from putting any thought into the next steps of my career.

I could have saved myself a lot of time and trouble if I had paused for a moment and made a list of challenges, benefits, and sticking points, like the one you're working on right now. Instead, once my on call time ended, I took the first job that came my way, and started a career path through misery. If I had made a list, or even considered my career from a personal and emotional viewpoint, I would have understood what makes me tick. Instead, I was still feeling the pressure of impressing everyone, doing a good job, and putting in a deathly amount of effort to prove my worth. (And I do mean deathly- I ended up being hospitalized with a severe case of bronchitis that I stoically ignored while I was trying to master a particularly tricky job duty.)

The idea of writing out why you want to work from home and how you got to this potential decision may seem silly or feel awkward, but it's the sort of uncomfortable exercise we all need to visit from time to time to truly understand what's on our mind and in our hearts. If I had known during that tumultuous time what I know now, I would've saved myself a good ten years of stress, heartache, headaches, and anxiety. My list would have looked something like this:

Why do I want to work remotely?

- My work environment is distracting due to a gossiping coworker who simply will not stop coming to my cubicle to tell me I'm going to get fired for some randomly perceived transgression.
- Coming to work at 7.30am is dangerous due to security not being on site until 9am.
- Scheduling meetings with East Coast and West Coast clients means no lunch break or dinner break- I'm working 7:30am to 8pm every day.
- I literally have no clean clothes because there's no time to do laundry.
- Since my manager works in another state and time zone, why do I need to be onsite?
- Due to VPN and laptop access, many of my job duties can be completed from any location with internet access.
- I spend the entire day in meetings about scheduling meetings. I could dial in to these meetings or skip them entirely so that I can focus on client-based tasks that are more urgent and more valuable for the company's bottom line.
- I have actually started to cry during rush hour traffic because I just want to be at home, in my pyjamas, eating a sandwich, in bed before I pass out for three hours and do it all over again.

As you can see, some of these items are perfectly rational, such as not wanting to walk through an urban location in the dark without security guards present. Other line items are things I need to work through on my own, like not having clean laundry. Others still are very much emotionally driven, like crying in traffic about a sandwich.

All of these items are valid, though. Every single item on this list inspired a new form of stress for me, to the point where I was so distracted by hating this routine, that I could barely take a deep breath and focus long enough to think about my actual tasks needing to be done. I was filled with a boiling resentment for all the things I needed to accomplish but couldn't.

At first, my list would have just said something like, "Because I hate it here and my life is in shambles and I don't know what to do." Only in a screaming, hysterical voice, because that's where I was emotionally.

Making this list is going to help you understand why you dislike your current job situation and help you discover that maybe you don't hate everything, after all. Unpacking your complicated thoughts and emotions that are urging you to work off-site will help you understand if that's what you really want, or if you just need to make some other personal changes in your life.

Maybe working from home or remotely is the best decision for you, but perhaps you just need a new job altogether. You might just need to simply sit down with your boss to discuss scenarios like your distracting coworker. The first step to understanding where you're headed is to create a list that includes every one of your problems- from the very real to the incredibly petty- that is pushing you away from the standard 8 hour office environment.

Chapter Three: The Pros & Cons of Working Remotely

After the previous exercise, you will likely be feeling one of three ways:
- More driven than ever to transition to working on the run
- Completely lost, confused, and possibly terrified
- Absolutely certain you'll never make this work

As someone who has made the transition myself, I will assure you that you will continue to feel these three waves of emotion throughout the rest of your career. Because there is absolutely no certainty in life, you can only do so much to prepare yourself for the endless barrage of "what ifs" that will surely come to surface. You'll at least be more aware of what you're looking at and have confidence in your ability to face the unknown.

The next step in preparing for a world far away from cubicles is identifying the pros and cons of working remotely. Again, these are not going to be the same for everyone and will probably be just as complicated as the first exercise. The overall goal of pinning down the benefits and challenges is to help you discover how truly plausible it is for you to work from another location. This will help you determine if you truly can use this method as an office escape.

To get you started, here are some of the most common pros and cons for working remotely sourced from my entire network of remote workers. This list encompasses freelancers, side-hustlers, crafters, and corporate telecommuters, and it is by no means reflective of every situation. This is just a little bit of inspiration to get you started on your own personal journey!

Pros	Cons
I can work from literally any location with a Wi-Fi signal	I've had to purchase/replace/service all of my own equipment
I don't have to spend two hours each day in my car	Sometimes I have to drop what I'm doing to go into the office for meetings/presentations
I don't have to change my lifestyle	I spend a lot more time on the phone than I did when I was in the office
Flexible hours- I log in when I want/need to	No social connection with my coworkers
Greater opportunities are available to me through freelancing	I have to discipline myself to complete all of my work on time
Since I'm not physically locked in meetings, I am more productive and present for my clients	My kids/pets think they need to sing or scream through every conference call
I get to spend more time with my family	Sometimes important information doesn't get to me, because it's discussed person-to-person in the office, and no one thinks to email me
I am far more productive without distractions	I have to be more creative and patient with myself when it comes to carving out time to work on very difficult/serious tasks

As you write out and discover your own personal pros and cons list, consider the weight you give to each item. For example, being able to work from any place with a WiFi signal was the most significant detail on my own personal list, whereas having to deal with my own equipment barely registered as being a negative thing. I would list my semi-functioning equipment as a "mild irritant," rather than a full-out "con." For you, however, that might be a huge impediment.

The same goes for distractions. I like to joke that Brad could complete a formal presentation through a full-blown hurricane, whereas I've been known to lose an entire hour because a butterfly landed on my hand. When you're working on your own, there will be both hurricanes and butterflies, on a literal and metaphorical level. Are you disciplined enough to keep yourself on track no matter what? Furthermore, is your job forgiving of these interruptions? For me, as a freelancer, I can simply add extra hours at the end of my day as needed, or continue writing a draft in a notebook. Brad, on the other hand, has to race to the nearest free WiFi spot any time our signal is interrupted, so that he can stay connected.

Your lifestyle is going to determine a lot of the pros and cons of working remotely. If part of the reason you're planning to change up your job situation is because your lifestyle is about to become radically different, add that to your pros and cons list, too.

In my situation, I had quit my job and lived on the road for quite some time before I started thinking about a new job. In that time, I did a lot of thinking about what I was going to do, and how I was going to make it work. Since my first transition, in which I put absolutely no thought into what I was doing, didn't turn out so well, I decided to put a lot of conscious effort into my new job. I did these exact exercises that I'm recommending to you now. In my experience, you can absolutely jump in the water and see if you can figure out how to swim before you drown, or you can learn about the mechanics of swimming before you approach the shoreline and give yourself a fighting chance of floating on safely.

Chapter Four: What Will You Accomplish With This Change?

There is one thing you need to know before we go any further with these exercises. You may still be thinking that working from home, the road, or your beachfront dreamhouse will allow you many hours of staring off dreamily into the distance. Perhaps you'll gain some time to do that, but let me assure you now:

If you want to slack off, this is not the workstyle for you.

No matter how hard you work in the office, you will still spend time taking breaks, chatting with coworkers, lingering over the coffee machine, walking up and down aisles to stimulate thoughts, having post-meeting rap sessions, and more. It's simply part of the office experience.

When you work from home, the stakes are higher, and the pressure is on. You are still expected to be on your A-game all day, but now there are distractions like you have never encountered before. Instead of having a walk-and-talk meeting to grab a cup of coffee with your manager, you'll find yourself walking with your laptop to the coffee maker so that you can continue your Skype conversation while you pour yourself that second cup of coffee you have desperately craved for the past two hours. Instead of dashing into the bathroom to check your appearance before an important meeting, you'll find yourself lecturing anyone who shares your home on the importance of staying completely quiet, even if there is an emergency, all while trying to coax your printer to unjam, and fielding a call from your coworker, who wants to know if you received the email she needs you to print out before the meeting.

It is very common for those who work outside of the office to report higher productivity, a greater focus on their work, and an unbelievable amount of output compared to when they had worked in the office. The difference, many hypothesize, is due to the level of discipline that we exercise when working from home, a van, a coffee shop, or our beachfront dream home.

At work, it's easy to give into distractions, because they're either tangentially work-related (that walk-and-talk to the coffee maker, for example), or they're your reward for doing something difficult (treating yourself to a sandwich from your favorite deli because you finished a report early, perhaps). Either way, any time you are in the office but not doing work, you still feel a sense that what you're doing is relevant to your job, and thus, you deserve to get paid for it.

It is extremely difficult to feel justified in getting paid for watching a butterfly sit on your hand for twenty minutes while you upload pictures of it to Instagram. You will absolutely feel more alive and connected to this planet, but if your boss or client asks why you dropped off a meeting abruptly, they are not going to be amused by butterfly pictures.

Perhaps there's a layer of guilt that drives those of us who work from our ideal location. Some say that expectations of remote workers are higher, because the jealous parties still in the office are hoping they'll fail. Likely, it's a little bit of both, along with the freedom from that burning anger or hopelessness that you felt in the office. Having more control and being at peace can be a miracle elixir for improving productivity.

The key part of that phrase, however, is "CAN BE." You know yourself better than anyone else. You know what you're capable of. You know how many mountains you can comfortably move each day. You know how much your kids, pets, partner, surroundings, etc will distract you.

In the next section of this book, we'll look at the different types of jobs that translate well to working remotely and working on the run. If you're thinking, "I can definitely handle the lifestyle, but not with my current job," then stick with this. We'll get there.

Maybe the opposite is true, and your current thoughts are, "Sure, my job would be ideal to take on the road, but I'm not sure I can wrap my head around stepping out of an office." No worries- there's a section for that too. Alternately, you might see the benefits and the possibilities, but the practicalities are way beyond your imagination. We'll definitely address those challenges, as well.

Before you put the effort into setting up a home office, before you hand in your resignation and take to the road, and before you admit out loud that you're interested in exploring the possibilities, you have to be real with yourself about your needs and what you want to get out of the experience.

I actually loved the job I quit in order to live on the road. I worked with a small group of people, and we loved each other like family. When I formally resigned, I used the phrase "it's not you; it's me" when talking to my boss. And while we laughed as I said it, it was true. I was not physically, mentally, emotionally, or psychologically intended to work from 8am to 5pm, Monday through Friday, regardless of what my work history indicated. Instead, I was born to work from when I get started to when I finish, 365 days a year.

Brad loves working. Brad loves working a little too much. While I might need an entire day to pause and refresh my brain, he doesn't turn off. When he worked at the office, I would have to call him around 8 or 9pm to remind him to come home. That's because when he's fully accessible to his staff and coworkers, he gets sucked into every single task that comes his way. I have seen him listen in on one meeting with his phone while being physically present in another meeting. Now that he works on the road, his focus is crystal clear. Sure, people still reach out to him 24 hours a day, but people can't appear in his space to distract him. He has become far more productive in far fewer hours.

I mention this to illustrate that there are many different ways in which taking your job on the road- even if it's just to your own home- can be an extraordinarily beneficial move. We'll go into this in more detail in a later section, but if you have spent the majority of your career working in an office, you will make a series of discoveries about yourself, your working method, your patience level, and more as you transition out of the office and into a solitary work style. The exercises I provide in this book are meant to gently ease you into this new reality, so that you don't find yourself in just as chaotic a situation as you found in the office.

Working from a location of your choice can help you control cost of living by allowing you to work in the town, state, country, or 1985 Volkswagen Vanagon of your choice. To a certain extent, working remotely gives you the opportunity to have full control over your work schedule, and what you accomplish in any given 24 hour period. You'll even have the ability to finally define what your time and your money mean to you, which will set you on the path to your ultimate career goals.

At the same time, acting upon this decision will require a great deal of discipline. You will face some uncomfortable truths about yourself. You will cry, you will fail, and you will have many awkward learning moments along the way. But, if you're willing to pick yourself up, dust yourself off, and head back to the drawing board a few times, armed with some constructive criticism and advice, you may be on the first leg of your journey to the work/life balance you've always dreamed of.

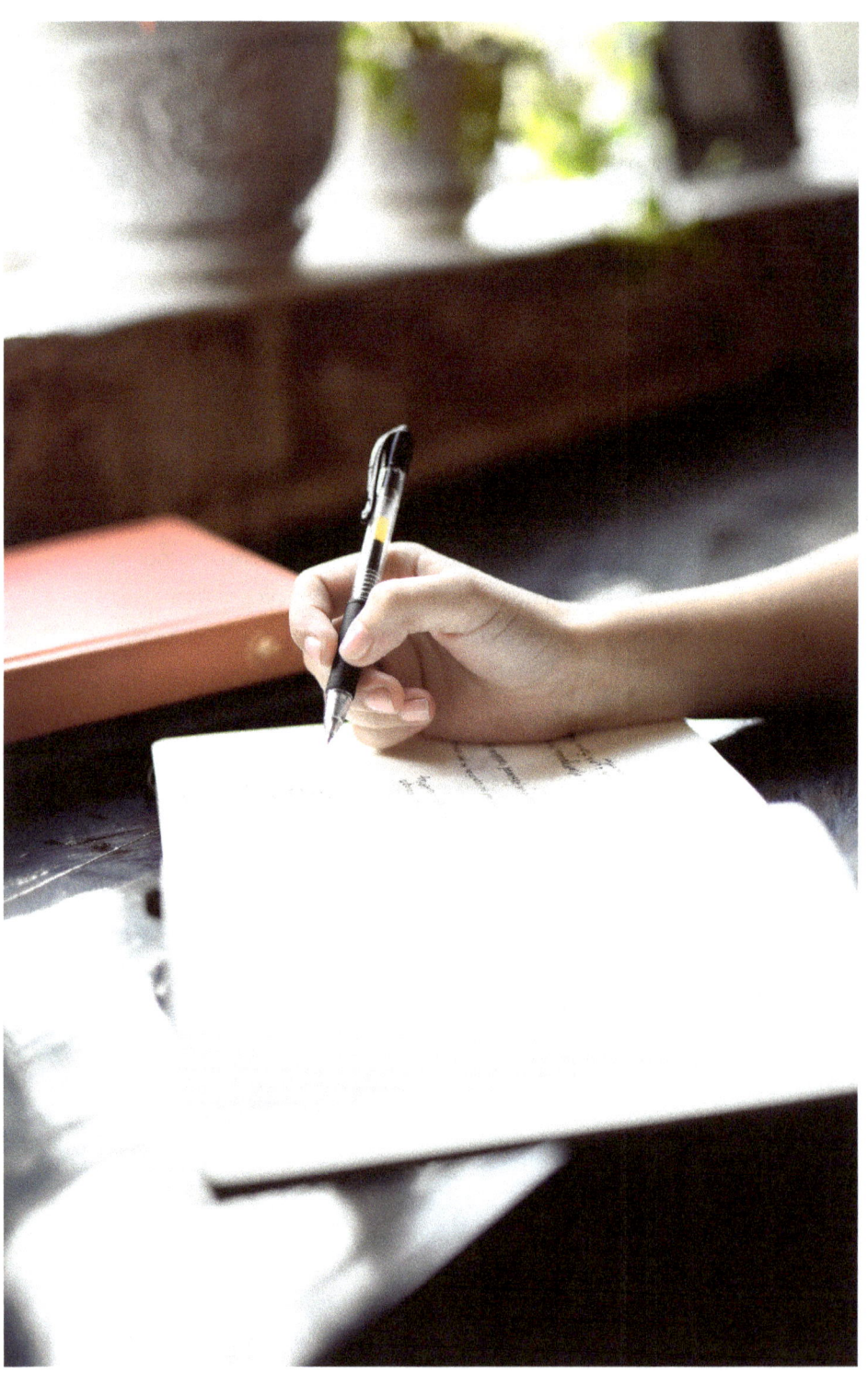

Section Two: Details, Details, Details

In the first section, we focused on exercises that will help wrap your brain around the why of wanting to take your work away from the office. Hopefully, that helped clarify some of the thoughts, emotions, and noise that has been buzzing around in your brain whenever you think about the topic of your career.

Now, you might be dealing with a different kind of buzzing- that of what your job is actually going to look like once you head out on your own. Are you interested in maintaining your current position, or something similar to it? Or are you ready to strike out on your own in a whole new area of expertise such as a freelancer, crafter, or hired hand? What types of skills are you willing to tap into, equipped to exercise, and can translate to the environment in which you're planning to work?

This is the time for hashing out details, and with that will come both answers to some of your current concerns, as well as a whole new batch of questions. Rest assured, that this book is intended to put you in the right position to answer all of those questions, even those which are exclusive to your current situation.

Chapter One: Determining the Who, Where, When, and How of Working on the Run

You are now in the Preliminary Stage of transitioning out of the office environment. This is the time to gather your resources and figure out what you want to do when you grow up, and how you plan to get to that point from here.

This journey may take a lot of directions. So far, you may not have considered the possibilities of a new job. As mentioned earlier, you might be perfectly happy with your current job and are willing to do what it takes to work with your employer to maintain the status quo, even if you're not physically present in the main office at all times.

Alternatively, you may have read the phrase "what you want to be when you grow up" and felt a spark of something inside. Maybe there's a certain inspiration that this transition could be a really big deal for you, as you finally go after that dream you've been harboring since you were a small child.

Anything is possible at this point in time, and it's up to you to decide what type of journey you're going to take here. In fact, it's time for another soul-searching, brainstorming session.

For this exercise, you might need a pen and some paper. You are going to go deep here, and ask yourself the one question that's going to set up the success of your transition from the office to the world. I recommend finding a quiet area, where you'll have minimal distractions and plenty of thinking space.

Your Challenge: An Exercise in Reality

The focus of this session is logistics: **How do you think this is going to work?** What comes to mind when you sit down and really think about working from the home, on the run, or anywhere in between?

Brad and I completed this exercise at different times, and our responses couldn't have been more different.

Brad actually started telecommuting about five years before we bought the van. Through a variety of job transitions, he found himself faced with the option to either move to Colorado, or start working from home. At the time, his family was a huge factor in our decision not to move, so he opted to set up a desk in the corner of our exercise room and started the process that way.

For Brad, there was little in the way of making the decision. Once he announced his plan to work from home, his company provided him with all of the equipment and technology necessary to move forward. They even sent him a fun desk organizer to congratulate him on his choice. His transition from working at home to van life was a bit more involved, but we'll cover that in more detail in the next section.

On the flip side, I had much more time to think about it, since I went from working full time in an office to living in a van with no transition. I started my journey of working on the run by daydreaming. In fact, I personally worked on this exercise a lot at night, staring up at the mosquito-speckled roof of the van, trying to quiet the panic that was rapidly rising every time I thought about "working" or "jobs."

I was equipped with a Creative Writing degree with the majority of my resume including writing as well. Ever since I was a child, the only thing I had really wanted to do was write, and I'd considered myself incredibly lucky that I had had multiple opportunities to flex that particular muscle throughout my seemingly-unrelated career in HR/Benefits and insurance. In fact, I'd gone on to pursue post-graduate certifications in various types of communications and marketing, so that I could do more writing, regardless of the position I held at the moment.

When I started daydreaming, I kept coming back to "what if I could write for a living?" So, on my mental map, I made that the start and end of all of my decision making. I was going to write. Now what was I going to write, and how was I going to find gigs was beyond me at this stage, and getting paid was a mystery that I hoped to solve sooner rather than later, but I had made up my mind.

Brad's and my situations represent just two of the ways you can look at this particular brainstorming session. You can stick with what you know, or you can go directly to manifesting your wildest dreams.

A visualization exercise is best for this quandary. Close your eyes, and picture yourself working. Are you seated at a laptop? Are you physically creating something? Are you in a quiet room, a noisy cafe, or surrounded by nature? What are your hands doing? What are your eyes looking at? Most importantly, how do you feel?

You're looking for a visual or daydream that makes you feel peaceful, alive, and productive. While there is not a single job I can think of that doesn't result in some form of cursing and wanting to throw everything out the window, that should not be the standard. In fact, for many, that's the reason you're completing this exercise in the first place.

So again, what does your new career look like? Is it the same thing, only in a different place? Or is it a brand new opportunity with horizons you haven't even begun to explore yet?

If these cerebral activities are starting to wear on you, I have good news: the next few exercises in this chapter are going to be purely objective. The next round of lists and brainstorming will be strictly fact-based, designed to help you manifest the reality that you just conjured in your visualizations.

Chapter Two: Who, Where, and When- Just the Facts

Even if you plan on doing this alone, know that you aren't really alone. You may be one person in an apartment, bungalow, van, skoolie, or yurt, but no one can have a career without someone to pay them.

That means you have to identify your connections and your network. If your aim is to continue your current job outside of the regular work boundaries, then your network will be fairly simple to identify. List everyone you require to make your job work. This can include:
- Your manager/supervisor
- Any superiors with whom you work directly on a regular basis
- Admins/support staff
- Schedulers
- Coworkers with whom you share projects or common duties
- IT/Tech Support
- Human Resources
- Benefits Helpline/ Employee Resource Center

You may also choose to reach out to others who work from home or telecommute that perform similar jobs to yours. They can act as mentors or at least springboards for any questions and thoughts you might have as your life quickly changes.

If you are going to continue to work your current job from a different location, you want to align yourself with connections that will help foster your productivity and keep you in touch with things that are happening inside the office. That can include anything from the latest water cooler discussions, to office gossip, or any underground rumblings about upcoming changes and projects.

For those who are thinking of spreading their wings elsewhere, you may already be feeling a little anxious about your network. First of all, know that you are not alone, either. When I started to feel drawn to a life of freelancing on the road, I lamented to Brad that I didn't know anyone who did this, and no one would ever understand me. As dramatic as that sounds, it felt like the truth to me. Going from a highly-structured corporate environment with timed bathroom breaks to a world where I simply have to deliver a quality product by a certain date is about as polar opposite as you can get in the working world. My friends- and even Brad- get second-hand anxiety when I tell them I took an afternoon nap, or that I ditched my manuscript for an early morning hike. It really seems like no one understands freelancers except for other freelancers.

Know that you are not alone. You are not the only person working on their own terms. Anyone who has a side-hustle, a personal business, or even someone who occasionally sells their creative works knows what you're going through. It doesn't have to be their full-time passion in order for them to appreciate your experience. These people are helpful connections.

So when you're making this list of your connections, be sure to include:
- People who own or have owned their own business
- Your friend who retired from corporate but now does pet portraits by commission only
- That person in the office who makes and sells soaps and lotions
- The person whom you've loosely connected to on social media

- who does freelance accounting
- Your nephew who makes several hundred bucks a month pet sitting
- Your chef friend who offers meal planning advice
- That guy you met at a bar who lives in a van and has the coolest Instagram ever

While your exact examples will surely differ, this group is about to become your biggest support network. Anyone who works independently with clients is going to be a wealth of information as you discover how to market yourself and your abilities. They may not understand all the elements of your particular situation, but these will be the people you call on when you need advice. When you suspect a client is trying to underpay you, you'll know who to contact. When you can't get a Wi-Fi signal even though everything is set up according to instructions, you'll know where to send a message for immediate help. If you're looking for an accountability buddy to prevent you from chasing butterflies for a few hours, these are the people who will know exactly what you mean by that and can coach you through a little self-discipline.

Now that you have your virtual team lined up, you need to size up the playing field. Location and surroundings have an incredible impact on anyone's ability to be productive and successful. The stress of the office environment might be one reason you're pursuing this option in the first place!

You will need to make sure that you have a designated work area, which we'll discuss in more detail later on. But for now, consider the following questions:
- Where will I work?
- Do I have adequate access to Wi-Fi, electricity, a phone signal, etc in this location?

If the answer to your first question is "in my home office," then you'll have no trouble with the second question. But if the answer to your first question is anything like mine- "in my van"- then the second question is answered with a solid "maybe?"

Those who are planning to truly work on the run need to strategize. Does your van/skoolie/RV have an adequate generator? Do you have decent Wi-Fi service nearly everywhere? Can you use your phone as a hotspot in an emergency?

In our case, Brad attends meetings almost all day, so he needs to have access to continuous phone signal and Wi-Fi. We have to be extremely strategic about staying "city-side" long enough for him to complete a work day, before we head out into the backcountry, where there might not be any sort of signal.

For many of us Van Lifers, this is a huge sacrifice, because we desperately want to be offline, off the grid, and somewhere wild and unrecognizable. If you haven't had the opportunity to drive across America, you may be surprised at how much of this country is completely un-wired. It's a beautiful sensation… until you can't send a client that file that's due at 9pm EST, you get dropped off of a phone call six times in a row, or you lose all of your edits because you didn't put your document on the cloud before you fell off the grid.

This is, unfortunately, the reality of working on the run. Though you want to be far from everything, there are some ties to the so-called "real world" that just cannot be severed. They can, however, be minimized by carefully selecting your location and being very deliberate in your scheduling.

This brings us to the "when" of working remotely. Regardless of whether your "where" is a spare bedroom or a converted school bus, you're going to need to know when you're working. Many people who leave the office find themselves working 24 hours, 7 days a week, 365 days per year. For the majority of the people who work this schedule, it is highly undesirable. It is an easy trap to fall into when you're not working in an office. Imagine you are knee-deep in a work project. As you type along, you don't notice the hours fly by, because you're completely engrossed. It's Thursday night, none of your programs are on. At some point, you stuff some cheese and crackers in your face because your stomach rumbles, but you keep working. There are no interruptions. Everything is great. Suddenly, you notice it's dark, so you glance down at the tiny clock on the bottom of your screen. 11:59pm. Seriously?

Pulling an all-nighter or an extra-long shift isn't unheard of in any industry. But it can easily become a habit when you don't have that social signal to get up, power down the computer, and go home. Your chair is cozy, your room is familiar, and all of the food and drinks you need are just a few steps away. While this can work for an extremely busy day, be careful about letting this become your usual schedule.

Humans need "on" time and "off" time. If your brain is constantly in performance mode, you will burn out very, very quickly. You will fail to enjoy anything that's going on around you, mostly because you don't notice it's happening. Your boss and team will come to expect you to be available 24/7, and you will resent them for this expectation. Work will become your life. Worst of all, you will potentially alienate everyone around you because you have made work your top priority and have placed everything else on the back burner.

I was headed down that path myself. When I first started freelancing, it was all too easy for me to work all of the time. I found myself getting up at 5am to start projects so I could have them submitted the same day. Unfortunately, my creative muses didn't appreciate this enthusiasm, and after a few weeks, I found myself completely unable to write. Words started looking strange. Amazingly, this confusion and extreme writer's block cleared up completely once I took a nice long nap, allowed myself some deep breaths and generous exercise, and took the opportunity to consume a few nutritious meals with the laptop closed.

Therefore, I strongly recommend that you exercise that control that you so crave by creating a schedule, even if you are not in a physical office. In the very first exercise of this book, we identified some of the reasons you wanted to work from home, and I mentioned that for nearly everyone, having control over your time and location is the number one factor. Now it is time to put that autonomy into effect.

Based on your sleeping habits, working through the night might be the best option for you. Or, if you have a lot of stuff to attend to, perhaps you schedule an "appointment day," where you allow yourself a few hours of time to take care of business, and make up those hours on other days. This can be extremely helpful for staying organized, since you'll know that any appointments you make will happen during that specific window of time, say, 8am to noon every Thursday. But best of all with this flexibility, you can take care of your own personal needs and develop your day around them.

Take a look at our schedules as examples of how this can work for you:

Brad	**Kristine**
Wake: Between 8am and 9am MST Immediately exercise a bit	Wake: At exactly 6:04am EST each morning Immediately exercise a bit
9:00am-10:00am: Make coffee, read emails, review previous day's projects	6.30am-10.30am: Organize files for the day and begin work
10:00am-2:00pm: Meetings, work, phone calls	10.30am-12:00pm: Eat and nap
2:00pm: Lunch	12:00pm-5:00pm: Continue Working
2:15pm forward: Continue working until falling asleep.	5:00-6:00pm: Close the laptop and call it a day.

There are, of course, exceptions to these schedules but generally speaking, this is what we adhere to. Brad's home office is on Mountain Standard Time, so he works on their schedule, regardless of where we are. None of my clients are in the same time zone, so I keep myself on Eastern Standard Time sheerly out of habit. Brad doesn't work on Saturday and Sunday, while I do, but typically only part of the day. Brad never sets an alarm, but I wake up to the same annoying noise every day at exactly the same time. These schedules are simply reflections of how we operate as people. I need something to get me up and motivated in the morning, or I'll stay in bed all day. I also need to specifically turn off by a set time, while Brad keeps going until he reaches a decent stopping point.

Looking at these schedules, which is more attractive to you? What is most reasonable for your job and work style? Do you have to be near a phone at specific times? Do you have tasks that need to be completed by a strict deadline? Are you a self-motivated kind of person, or do you drizzle your way from task to task as the mood strikes?

Again, some of these are pretty philosophical questions, and you'll most likely find yourself changing your mind a few times as you try to hit your stride. Early in my freelancing career, I received an email from an angry client who was perturbed that I didn't answer her Skype calls at 3am. "Aren't your type supposed to be up and available all hours of the day?" she asked. I spent a significant amount of time wondering if I should be. After all, this was my career of choice- shouldn't I live up to the standards of my job? Ultimately, I decided the care of my own mental, physical, and emotional health- all of the things that I took into consideration when I transitioned out of the office and on my own- were more important than answering emails at 3am, so I simply replied, "I am available between 8am and 6pm, EST." And with a few exceptions, that has been true ever since.

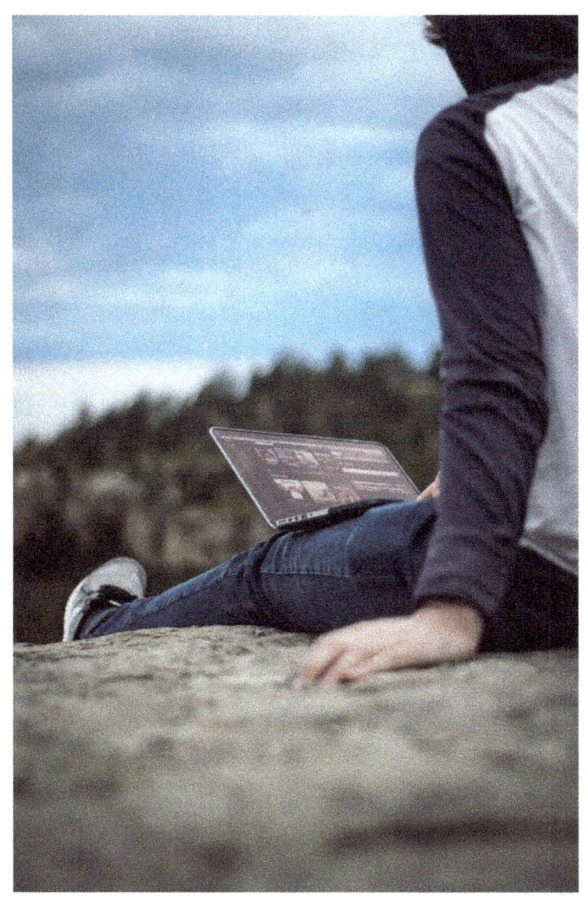

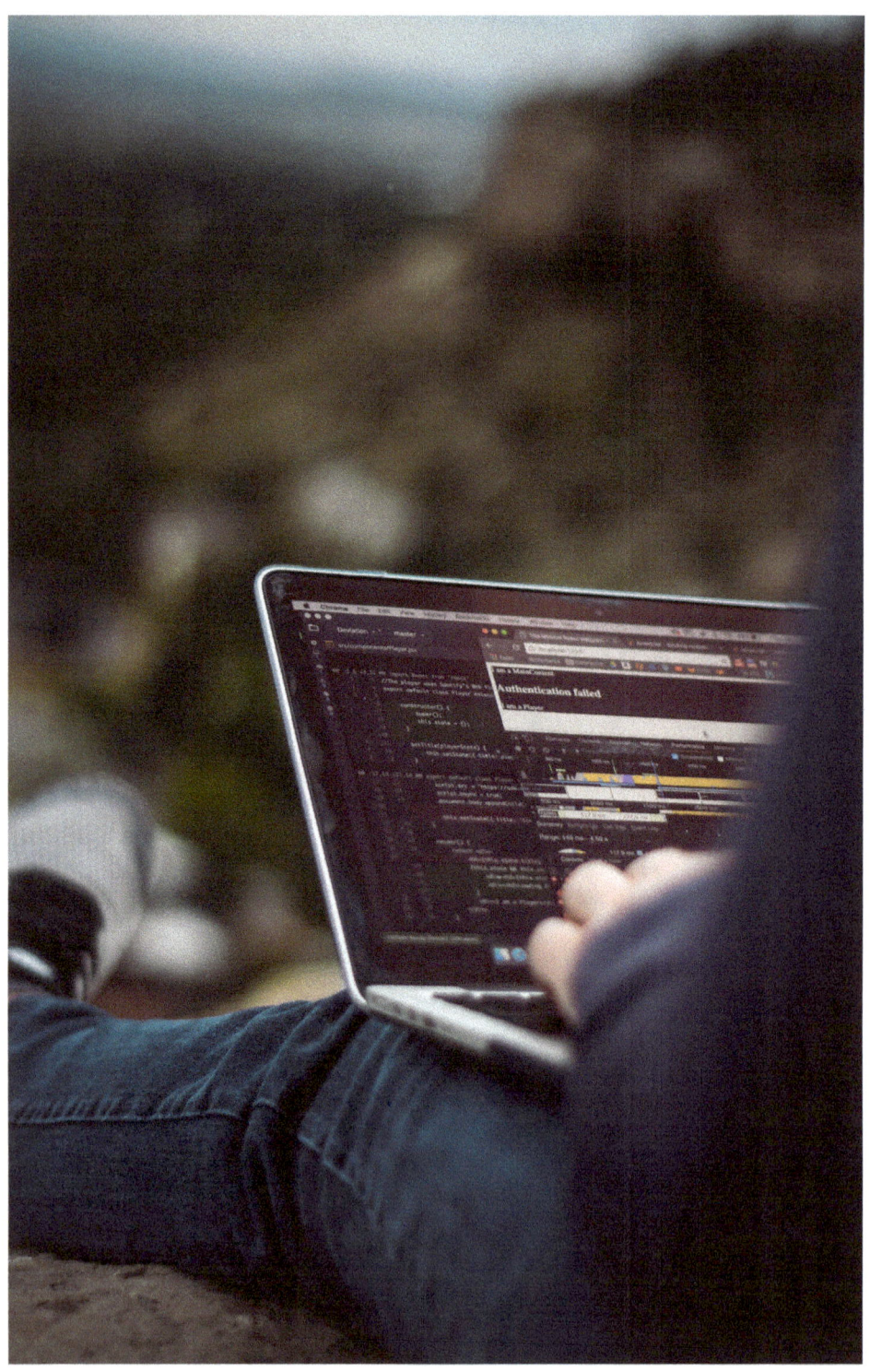

Section Three: What Will I Be? What Will I Do?

So far, we've focused a lot on logistics. For some of you, this means that you're feeling more focused than ever, with a renewed sense of resolve to make this whole thing happen. Others still might feel a lot of apprehension, with thoughts such as, "It's great that I know my support network, but I don't even know what my job is going to be, or if I'm going to be able to afford to live!"

Those are valid concerns. Here's the thing when it comes to changing your lifestyle completely: It can be done immediately, but you will feel so much more prepared if you have taken the time to reflect on your resources, your needs, and your goals. When my division was sold, and I found myself suddenly jobless, one of the most uttered phrases at the resulting "Unhappy Hours" was "I just wish I'd been prepared." This is your chance to make a bid for greatness. Assuming you aren't already in a jobless position, you have all the opportunity you need to get your ducks in a row first.

Or maybe you have already been let go, or in an inspired moment, told your boss you're going to go live in a van. I've been there, as well. There are a lot of ways we can get to this point- some are positive, and some are not so pleasant. Some of you are about to be the happiest you've ever been. Even more of you are going to use this experience as a springboard to something more amazing than ever.

In this section, we're going to look at different jobs, and put them to the "on the run" test. There are some jobs that make absolutely no sense as WFH or van life jobs. However, if that is your field, you can still make this van lifestyle work.

The next several chapters are going to introduce various opportunities. Some of them may not feel as if they are relevant to your specific situation, but I encourage you to read the chapter anyway (or at least give it a healthy skim). There will be some tips, words of wisdom, and things anyone can consider in each section.

Chapter One: Same as It Ever Was

Brad loves his job. What he actually does is very technical and involved, but essentially, he provides support and client interfacing in software development for a global firm. Brad has always loved his job, and it shows. He is available 24/7, phone signal permitting. Brad once gazed across a canyon, observing the beauty of Bandelier National Monument while chatting about eligibility files with his team. He is dedicated to his job at a level that I personally consider unhealthy, but his job brings him great joy, so this works for him.

Brad's original plan was to quit his job. He had already been working from home, but we both agreed that it would be hard to live in a van with no plan or itinerary, while balancing an intensive full time job. So he gathered his management team, and calmly explained to them that he and his wife had decided they needed to live in a 1985 Volkswagen Vanagon and that he wanted to leave by this date. He let them know that they would need to carve out an exit strategy.

I wasn't there for the phone call, or the rest of the afternoon, but I was very anxious to hear how it went. Brad seemed off when he came downstairs at the end of the day, but I couldn't put my finger on what was wrong. He explained that his management team had told him that they really needed him, and after spending the day consulting with various corporate leaders, they had offered him a six month leave of absence with benefits, as well as a bonus if he returned to work on a specific date.

I personally love telling this story, because it goes to show that this type of job transition doesn't have to be a negative thing. You may be greatly surprised by how accommodating your employer is, if you approach the potential movement of your work space from a very practical and positive space.

When having these types of discussions with others in your workplace, it is beneficial for everyone involved if you are organized and have taken the time to prepare with a few notes about your own needs and goals identified.

We touched earlier on productivity, which is often at the forefront of every manager's mind. For the most part, the location of your actual body doesn't matter to your team so much as that you are actively working, meeting deadlines, and getting the job done. Therefore, before you start discussions with your boss, I encourage you to explore this topic with yourself, and to do so very honestly. It's easy to say "sure, I'm productive!" Take a look at all of your notepads in the office. Are they filled with work-related notes and productive efforts, or are they more grocery lists, calculations for your own bills, daydreams, and things that demonstrate you're not really attending meetings on a mental level? Reflect on your performance reports. Do they advise you to look into time management courses?

If self-discipline, motivation, and staying on task aren't your most valuable skill set, that's okay. In fact, many people find that working from home removes a lot of distractions. For example, you won't be able to wander the aisles of your office, looking for someone who wants to chat. You won't be tempted to walk down to the cafeteria for a superfluous cup of coffee because there are no sympathetic cafe workers for you to laugh and joke with, rather than hurrying back to the office.

Then again, maybe it's not the people that are the distraction. Maybe you're so done with your coworkers that you spend most of the day listening to music. If anyone knew how much time you spent looking up lyrics and re-playing sick drops, they'd probably take your audio card away, but as far as anyone can tell, you're over there typing away. Or it could be your phone and the world of social media that has you grasped in its talons of constant conflict and gossip. Will these temptations intensify when you work from a place where you can have constant access to anything you want?

For most people, that's not a situation they can accurately predict. You need to be able to critically look at your work style and identify HOW you get things done. Then you need to plan some actions that will help you with your focus, so that you can be productive.

I have always been a procrastinator. I'm famous for coming in with that eleventh hour Hail Mary for the win when it came to huge projects in the corporate setting. At the same time, I have always shown up, ready to work, and never neglected even the most trivial daily duties, like watering the office plants. This is why I get up so early. At 6:04am, hardly anyone in my network is posting on social media. My European friends are at work. My Australian and Asian buddies are ending their days, and no one else in my hemisphere is awake to text and chat with me. Brad is still asleep, so I can't torment him. The most distracting thing that happens in the morning is each glorious sunrise (weather permitting), and I absolutely allow myself a few quiet moments to enjoy that part of the day.

Generally speaking, though, that sets me up for a productive day. By the time Brad is awake and encroaching on my coffee supply, I'm already in work mode. There have been times I've had to hide my phone from myself. Sometimes I put on headphones and listen to binaural tones, because if I listen to anything with lyrics and a beat, I'm going to have a personal dance party. You have to know yourself so that you can figure out what needs to be done to rein yourself in.

Ask yourself a series of questions:

1. What is my go-to distractor? This could be social media, games on your phone, music, etc.

2. What is it that this distraction gives me? Perhaps it's social interaction, or maybe a mental break.

3. What happens if I try a more productive type of break? Consider closing your eyes and taking ten deep breaths, or getting up from your workstation, having a few sips of water, and returning. Sometimes you really do need to tune out for a minute, to refocus.

This confidence in your productivity is what will project to your manager and Human Resources team. In your early conversations, don't let productivity be an elephant in the room. Empathize with their concerns and demonstrate that you have already considered this, and that you've already taken measures to address this possible challenge.

Hand-in-hand with productivity comes practicality. Specifically, will you be available for the amount of time your job needs you, and within the typical working day? In some situations, such as the example mentioned earlier in which you need to make regular appointments, the hours you work will definitely need to change. This could be due to any number of things, including needing to drop kids off at school or daycare at a certain time, medical appointments, or even a reduction in weekly hours for your physical or mental health, etc.

Your employer is likely going to be concerned that you won't be able to meet deadlines adequately. Think of ways you can be transparent with your manager early on so that this is less of a worry. As time goes by, you'll prove through your actions that you're still productive and efficient, but at first, your team will worry that you're out there chasing butterflies with people like me, instead of getting work done. You can offer to create a project list, or use a time-tracking software to help put them at ease. It might make you feel micromanaged, but if you're focused and determined, there's really nothing to fear.

When discussing this with your employer, make sure you approach it through the lens of collaboration. Let your team know that you appreciate that this is going to be a huge change for your office group as well as yourself. Think of things you can do to ease the burden for all of you, and bring those up in your talks with your manager. Let your employer know your specific availability, and actually plan to show up at those times.

Employers want to know that you are going to be just as valuable when you aren't under their watchful gaze. Consider- and then share with them- your thoughts on the practicality of working off-site. If there is a particular job duty that would be a fantastic opportunity for your skillset offsite, bring that up, as well.

For example, in one client relationship management position, our group had to run a specific report for all clients each Friday. This report was massive and because it included so much information, it would lock up your laptop for hours, which essentially rendered you useless for completing any other tasks- including speaking to clients. Coincidentally, anyone who didn't have major meetings on Fridays was permitted to work from home. One Friday, as I was wrapping things up in my at-home office, I offered to run the report. Imagine how many lightbulbs went on with my team when I was able to send everyone the report results after a few hours, and no one lost productivity (in fact, I got a load of laundry done and started dinner). From then on, the report was run as the last task of the day by someone who was working from home.

This is the sort of innovation that can make the concept of working outside of the office look very appealing to all parties involved. Sure, you may have to take on a regular task that was previously shared, but as a compromise, you're also getting the freedom to work from anywhere, with the added bonus of a more flexible schedule.

Once you have your working hours settled, and your team has discussed a practical and reasonable approach to meeting all of your regular deadlines and maintaining productivity levels, it's time to get into the less subjective details.

The first thing to get out of the way is who is paying for what expenses. In many cases, your company will set you up with a laptop and other equipment. Depending on your industry, they might want the laptop to have certain specifications, drivers, and programs, which they'll want to install through internal tech support. You'll need to think about monitors, printers, a mouse, a keyboard, and any other supplies you deem necessary.

You'll also want to look into options regarding your telephone. Depending on your job, an employer will provide you with a specific phone to be used strictly for work purposes. Other employers are willing to foot your entire monthly phone bill or at least part of it if you use it for work. Many larger corporations have access to discounts from major cell phone providers, so this tends to work out well for everyone involved.

As you iron out these technological details, make sure you know where your tech support will come from. It's easy enough to jog down to IT to ask a quick question or to get more batteries for your mouse now, but when you're not working in the office, who do you call? Who pays for the batteries? Furthermore, does that company-issued cell phone have service where you're headed? If you have a problem with the phone, do you head to the provider's local retail shop, or call someone within your company? Knowing these things before they happen in the mountains of Idaho or somewhere deep within the Ozarks is crucial.

One sensitive subject that needs to be addressed is your total compensation package. If you're receiving benefits such as medical, dental, and vision insurance now, are those benefits contingent on the number of hours worked or on your work location? If so, what options are available for you to continue those benefits? Are you still eligible for time off if you're not physically in the office? That can include time off due to illness or injury, as well as any vacation time. Will you still accrue or receive time off allowances at the same rate? What about disability pay?

Another concern may be job protection under the Family Medical Leave Act (FMLA) or state-mandated leaves, such as maternity and paternity leaves. If part of the reason you're changing your job situation is to care for yourself or a family member who has medical needs, you'll definitely want to be sure that those types of protection are still extended to you if you work remotely.

At first, you might think that it will be simple to just pick up your job and move it to your house, your van, or any place you might prefer to work. However, once you start thinking more about logistics, you'll discover there's a lot more to it than the location of your laptop. Having open and frank discussions with your management team and Human Resources department will help you think about all the minutiae that are often taken for granted in an office environment.

Still, this is not an impossible task. Start by focusing on the main topics of productivity, practicality, and the day-to-day details. At first you may have to make compromises which benefit the company. Try hard to keep an open mind and appreciate the concerns your employer may have. Understand who you are as a worker, but also how you fit into the organization as a resource. You may fear that your manager doesn't "trust" you, but ultimately, the concerns they may have about your productivity and the practical aspects of your transition off-site are less personal, and more about the organization as a whole. Let them know you plan to be there 100 percent in mind and effort, just not in body, and the conversation will certainly be more positive.

Chapter Two: Redefining the "Free" in "Freelancing"

For some reason, when most people think about freelancing, they immediately think of writing, journalism, and photography. That's not entirely incorrect; in fact, those are the most popular outlets of freelancing. However, contract work and consulting is available in all sorts of fields. Whether those positions are something you can incorporate into your lifestyle, though, is something you'll have to fully explore before you commit time or money.

For someone who lives in a van, I'm incredibly risk-averse. I enter the literal and proverbial water one toe at a time, and when I started considering the possibilities of freelance copywriting, I approached it very, very slowly. I started with lots of research. Every time Brad was behind the wheel, I would look up various temporary writing gigs. I read everything I could on the topic, from online magazine articles, to Reddit postings from people who currently freelance. I wanted to know what the experience was like before I jumped in.

Most people will find that this is a good move, because expectations and reality are rarely aligned when you first start working on your own. You will need to establish personal boundaries, but you need to make sure that the hard lines you draw are reasonable for what you want to do. When I implemented my strict availability guidelines, for example, I made myself ineligible for a lot of great gigs that would have been perfect for me... if I was willing to work until I literally keeled over. There will be a lot of situations in which you will have to uncomfortably say "no," but in each of these scenarios, it's necessary to do so.

So I urge you to start the freelance job hunt slowly and methodically. Read the horror stories. Look at the job postings. Don't get sucked in by the ads that promise you'll make six figures a year doing what you love. You can, of course, if you spend all of your time working, but van lifers especially don't like that concept. From the statistics to the anecdotes, read it all.

Then it's time to get to work on organizing yourself.

First, think about your talents and skill sets. What can you do that is marketable? Nearly everything can be turned into a freelance gig. I know accountants, dietary consultants, illustrators, videographers, photographers, personal assistants, telemedicine nurses and therapists, lifestyle and health coaches, and travel agents, all of whom can take their job wherever they care to be at any given time. If you need help getting ideas, take a look at popular freelance networking sites, like Fiverr or Upwork. Look at the different categories and postings, and get an idea where your niche is.

Next, look at the time you want to dedicate to these opportunities. If working a regular eight-hour workday is something you hope to continue, then go for it. If you want to have your days free, then work at night. For most gigs, the actual timing within the day doesn't matter as much as meeting deadlines and being available to communicate. Other gigs have specific time-related requirements. For example, photographers require a certain amount of light in order to shoot properly, and personal assistants need to be on the ball with deadlines.

Equipment is also an important thing to factor into this decision. If you're going to be sending lots of files, you'll want to make sure that your computer can handle a lot of data, and/or cloud access. If you're going to be creating a lot of visuals, you'll need cameras, tablets, illustrator programs, and editing software to bring your ideas to life.

Every job requires a variety of resources, and you'll need to make sure those are available to you, especially if you're going to be mobile. If your plan is to work from your home, storage is not as much of an issue. But when you're working from the road, space is a huge consideration. Will being on the road hinder your workflow? Will it limit what you can do because you don't have space for the equipment? Now is the time to think critically about the logistics and what is actually feasible for you.

Finally, you need to be brutally honest with yourself about income. I wish I could tell you that all freelancers are filthy rich, and that we just keep working because we're dedicated to our craft. I'm sure there are a few who are, but I have yet to hear a "getting started in freelancing" story that doesn't sound like the typical "young actor moving to the city" tale.

When you first appear on the scene, you can be Nobel Prize level talented, but you'll still need to network. You'll need to create a name for yourself. That means taking on the little tiny jobs that will prove that you actually have a scrap of talent. Over time, these clients will (hopefully) ask you to take on projects that are slightly larger in scope, and you'll get more credit, more money, and earn a better reputation.

Ask any small business owner from your list of contacts in Section Two. The first few years are going to be rough as you establish yourself. Working with a contracting site like Fiverr or Upwork can potentially speed up this process, but there will be stipulations and contracting fees involved.

You may land a glorious gig right off the bat, but that doesn't mean the work will always be there. My third contract was a long-term, high budget project for a real estate firm. It was a beautiful experience, but the contract eventually ended. That's simply the reality of freelance work- it is not a permanent position, and you will have to constantly hustle to find new gigs.

Can you afford this lifestyle? Will you be comfortable without the certainty of a paycheck? Are you pretty good with saving money for a rainy day? If your ideal scenario is to only work when you have to, then freelancing is perfect for you. But if you need to have a $2000 paycheck every other Friday in order to feel comfortable, then you may want to re-examine this option.

Hand-in-hand with pay come the other parts of compensation, such as benefits, taxes, and time off. These are very real parts of the working experience, at least in the United States, and you won't be exempt from needing medical and dental care or from paying taxes just because you're sitting in a van or skoolie. Research what options are available to you before you make the plunge, and get a feel for the tax requirements before you find yourself in a bind. There are plenty of materials out there to help freelancers find their feet, some of which I've included in the "Resources" section at the end of this book.

Freelancing can be incredibly rewarding, and the whole "free" part of it makes it ideal for folks who aren't made to work in a traditional office setting. Plus, technology has advanced to the point that it is now easier than ever to connect with others who are looking for your specific set of skills and talents.

Just remember, nothing comes truly for free. You will have to hustle. You will have to put yourself out there. The work is hard, and oftentimes you'll look back at your corporate paycheck with nostalgia and longing. But if that control factor is truly at the heart and soul of your decision to take your work on the run, freelancing is a great fit!

Chapter Three: A Side-Hustle You Can Do All Day- or Not!

Side-hustles are the latest phenomenon amongst the working population, and it's easy to see why. These are the fun-sized versions of jobs, so to speak. Not only do you get to choose a money-making process that is fun and enjoyable for you, but you can work as much or as little as you want.

You can turn nearly any type of task into a side hustle, depending on your skills and interests. If you're a crafty or creative type, those talents can translate into a side-hustle very easily. As an example, one friend of mine is a very talented seamstress, and she has made an impressive living for herself doing basic mending and repairs as she and her husband travel in their big rig RV from campsite to campsite throughout the year. Another friend charges $5 per animal to walk dogs and keep pets entertained from her massive skoolie.

Coming up with a side-hustle may require a bit of creativity on your part, but everyone has a marketable skill. Side-hustles aren't necessarily tied to van life, either, anyone with the desire to can do them.

To come up with your side hustle, you need to look deep into your passions, and find a talent you enjoy that's profitable. I wrote an entire book about this process, called "How to Choose the Ultimate Side-Hustle: Making Money and Being Your Own Boss," but I'll lay out the groundwork here so you can decide if this is an option you'd like to pursue.

Similar to freelancing, there are nearly infinite opportunities that make ideal side-hustles. Here are just a few different niches and options that you might consider:

Type of Hustle	Examples
Creative	home made arts and crafts, such as knitting or needlework, woodworking, painting or drawing, ceramics, jewelry making, quilting, soap making or creating bath goods, teaching crafting/creative classes,
Resale	rehab/refurbish of furniture, clothing, collectibles, vintage ware
In-person	pet sitting, housecleaning, babysitting, tutoring, pet grooming, car washing, yard work, drive for Uber/Lyft or a food delivery service, mystery shopping
Online help	tutoring, resume writing, affiliate marketing, email marketing, virtual assistant, blogging, drop shipping

Some of these are going to work best if you plan on working from a stationary location, but you might be surprised at what you can take on the road. I know a woman who makes a small fortune in resale, and she's been living the van life for ten years. In fact, she attributes her success to her ability to travel anywhere, because she can accumulate collectibles and trinkets all over the country, knock the dirt off of them, and sell them via her website. She has her methods of storing them, taking good photographs, and then it's just a matter of keeping track of stock and shipping them as they sell.

Taking a side-hustle on the road does have a special set of considerations, as this example shows. She needs to make sure nothing is damaged so that she can sell the items and make money. That may seem impossible when you're on the road, since vans aren't usually climate controlled, and are generally in motion, jostling down bumpy roads. She has a system involving a padded drawer, towels, and plenty of bubble wrap. While you may not want to take on huge furniture restoration projects on the road, you might have a great time turning t-shirts into teddy bears. Let your mind wander a bit and see how creative you can truly be.

Having an in-person side-hustle while living on the road is another place where you might get stuck in the logical considerations, but it's not impossible. All across the country, you can find huge campgrounds where many part-time wanderers make their seasonal homes. These parks are filled with families, children, and pets. A babysitter or tutor would take a lot of stress off of parents' minds if they'd like to have some alone time. Watching their dogs will leave them free to explore places where Fido might not be welcome. And what harried mother wouldn't enjoy having someone else deep-clean their camper while they enjoy a few moments of peace and quiet? Even if you're just parked for a few nights, making your services known can bring in some spare cash quickly.

Online side-hustles are one place where road warriors can truly shine… as long as they have access to a good Wi-Fi connection! While people have been using the internet to make money since the early days of Angelfire, many of the options mentioned in the previous table are fairly new types of online gigs. Tutoring and resume writing are pretty familiar opportunities, but now there is newer video conference technology, like Zoom and Skype, that have changed how online courses and tutoring sessions are conducted. A virtual assistant gig is very much similar to that of a personal assistant- only with all communication taking place over text, chat, teleconferencing software, or email.

Affiliate and email marketing, as well as drop-shipping and blogging are definitely some examples of phenomena that have only appeared in recent internet history. Though each of these can be a side-hustle of its own, many people combine a little bit of each craft to create their own brand.

Affiliate marketers are hired by larger, online-based companies to essentially do their marketing for them. Rather than hiring professional ad departments and high price-tag marketing gurus (or sometimes in addition to), these companies hire regular everyday folks to come up with an ad campaign. That means you'll choose ad space, banners, and find interesting ways to capture the attention of the public, on behalf of the larger company. In exchange, they'll give you a personal marketer code, so that when anyone clicks on your ad to purchase their products, you will get a commission from the sale. Some of these affiliate marketing opportunities can be incredibly lucrative, especially when high-ticket items like cars, boats, or vacations are at stake!

Email marketing combines a bit of copywriting, a bit of marketing, and a bit of tech know-how. If you've purchased anything online, you've probably gotten at least one or two email follow-ups from that particular vendor. Email marketing is incredibly popular and effective, with sales and special offers coming to our inboxes all the time. In this gig, you'll be tasked with coming up with attractive copy and procuring a list of dedicated subscribers, which is usually provided to you. You then make sure the communications go out regularly, do any cleanup of unsubscribers or failed email addresses, and review the open rates and effectiveness of your campaigns. You may be asked to try different marketing approaches to increase appeal, and in some cases, tasked with responding to inbound email.

Drop-shipping is a very interesting approach to having your own online retail store, and an option that I'm seeing more and more frequently as a side hustle both in and out of the van community. In this model, you set up an online store- a website where you sell... stuff. Anything you can think of. You market your goods, attract customers and so on. But when people buy your "stuff," it's actually coming from a third party supplier- usually the manufacturer. You don't have to make anything, nor do you have to ship anything. All you have to do is set up the website, bring in the customers, and make sure they're happy.

And last- but certainly not least- there's blogging. This concept isn't new, but the idea that you can get paid for musing at length about a specific topic is still somewhat of an innovation. Bloggers get paid through selling ad space on their blogs, finding sponsors, and quite often with a touch of affiliate marketing.

There is a very blurry line- if any at all these days- between "social media influencers" and "bloggers." You can test this phenomenon by looking up a recipe. Any recipe will do! You'll likely find someone's food blog, where they'll meander through a touching story, followed by their experiences preparing this dish, complete with pictures and step-by-step detailed instructions. As you read, you'll notice that they mention very specific brands for some ingredients. That's the ticket to getting paid.

As a van lifer, you have a very particular niche at your fingertips when it comes to blogging and/or social media influencer potential. Our lifestyle is pretty unique, and setting up social media accounts, blogs, and websites is a typical practice in our community. Not only is it a great way to keep in touch with our friends and family back home and around the world, but it's the easiest way to save memories and photos of our journeys. I would be lying if I said I didn't occasionally have to peek at Brad's journal or my own blog to remember a certain location where we camped, or to double-check a particular hike to make sure I correctly recalled the spot.

There are ways to monetize your van life blog or social media account, such as checking in with potential sponsors and running some ads. You might also have a devoted group of followers who would love to purchase merchandise with your van name, blog handle, or logo printed on it!

To be perfectly clear, you do not have to be a van lifer to run a successful blog or social media account. There are plenty of lifestyle topics that are interesting and read well on blogs. You can even write a blog about how you transitioned from working in an office to working at home!

When it comes to choosing a side-hustle, innovation and strategy are key. It is rare to find success overnight. In fact, you'll likely have to work harder at finding followers, customers, and clients than you would as a freelancer. That being said, nearly everyone loves their side-hustle and wouldn't trade it for the world, though it's very simple to step away from a side-hustle when it no longer serves you!

Chapter Four: Here, There, and Everywhere

You've probably seen an older television show or movie, in which a character proclaims to be "just traveling through" and "looking for some odd jobs" while they're in town. Like me, you might have thought that this was some old-fashioned ideal from days when the nomadic lifestyle was relatively popular, with folks riding the rails or even a horse out West to see what they could rustle up. In reality, this is still common amongst van lifers and explorers!

When it comes to living in a van, skoolie, RV, or any type of home on wheels, most people find themselves feeling a little disoriented by constantly moving. They'll find a spot to park for awhile, so they can get their bearings, along with a nice, hot shower and some clean laundry. Brad and I have done this many times- sometimes not on purpose, such as when the van has required extensive repairs. It provides a nice change of pace when you get to know a town or area a little bit before moving on.

Some people park cyclically in order to make a quick living before moving on. They'll find a reasonable location to park or camp, or even take up a bed in a hostel for a bit. Then, they'll find a temporary job for a month or even a few months, earning a regular paycheck and saving as much money as possible. After some time, with their financial stores replenished, they'll hit the road again.

There are quite a few jobs that lend themselves well to this lifestyle, such as seasonal warehouse and industrial work. Many temporary placement agencies are thrilled to have a reliable worker on hand for a short period of time. There's no pressure on anyone to find a long-term assignment, which can be beneficial for an employer who just needs someone to fill in while another person is on leave, or during peak season.

All of these types of positions will provide training, but some require a specific skill set that can make you a valuable asset as you seek out these temporary shifts. For example, warehouse or industrial jobs might require someone who is certified to drive a forklift or operate specialized equipment. Not everyone has those skills on their resume, so you'll be an instant hire if you show up in a new town with these types of qualifications.

Depending on how long you feel comfortable staying in one spot, these types of contracts can be very rewarding, both monetarily and through the contacts and experience you'll gain. I have a few young male friends who pop up at various warehouses across the country. They love how picking, stocking, and machine operating all day for a few months can keep them in peak shape, while padding their bank accounts for their next big adventure.

There are a few things to keep in mind when looking into these options, however. First, most temporary positions will require you to sign a contract for a specific period of time. While many states are "at will" employers, meaning you or the employer may terminate your contract for any reason and without warning, these contracts will make you stay put for a while. If you're not comfortable with looking at the same streets for more than a few days, this might not be the right fit for you.

Then there's the exact opposite issue: you might get attached. I had the opportunity to watch this play out with one of my college buddies. He bought the van and traveled. He stopped in a town in New Mexico to do some odd jobs. He met a very nice young lady. He and his wife are now permanent residents of a town in New Mexico.

On the other hand, I have several friends who have made the conscientious decision to not get attached. They prefer to be as brief as possible in order to avoid a mishap in which they find themselves permanently settled in a single location, at least for the time being. This is a perfectly valid narrative as well, so long as you are fully aware of what type of personal situation you want to maintain.

Lastly, it's very important to be clear to your employers that you are not in this for the long haul. You want to set up the expectation that you will be on hand as long as the contract allows, and then you will be gone. If you've got a terrific work ethic and knock it out of the park on all of your duties, the employer may try to coax you to stay longer, but that choice is entirely yours. You don't want to give anyone false hope that you're going to stick around, or pin you for a promotion when there are long-timers who may also deserve those opportunities.

Chapter Five: Something for Everyone

As you can see, there's a little bit of everything available to those who work from home, on the road, or anywhere in between. Yes, adapting a specific job to your preferred remote situation may require a little finesse and creativity. There will be some research involved, some planning, and some strategy to get all of the moving pieces to fit just right.

Now that you've reviewed some options and examples of careers that can be taken anywhere, and professionals who make their jobs, work wherever they go, the brainstorming exercises from the first section might be making a little more sense. In order to be successful while doing your work on the run or even from your home office, you need to be thoroughly grounded in reality while constantly having your creative brain on in case you need to troubleshoot or find a solution to a problem you've never had before.

Even if nothing about your job changes at all, the situation is going to be very different. The problems will be new, and even solutions to familiar challenges will require a different outlook. But, if you're mentally prepared for what lies ahead, adapting to change and overcoming obstacles while still being productive will be the ultimate version of success!

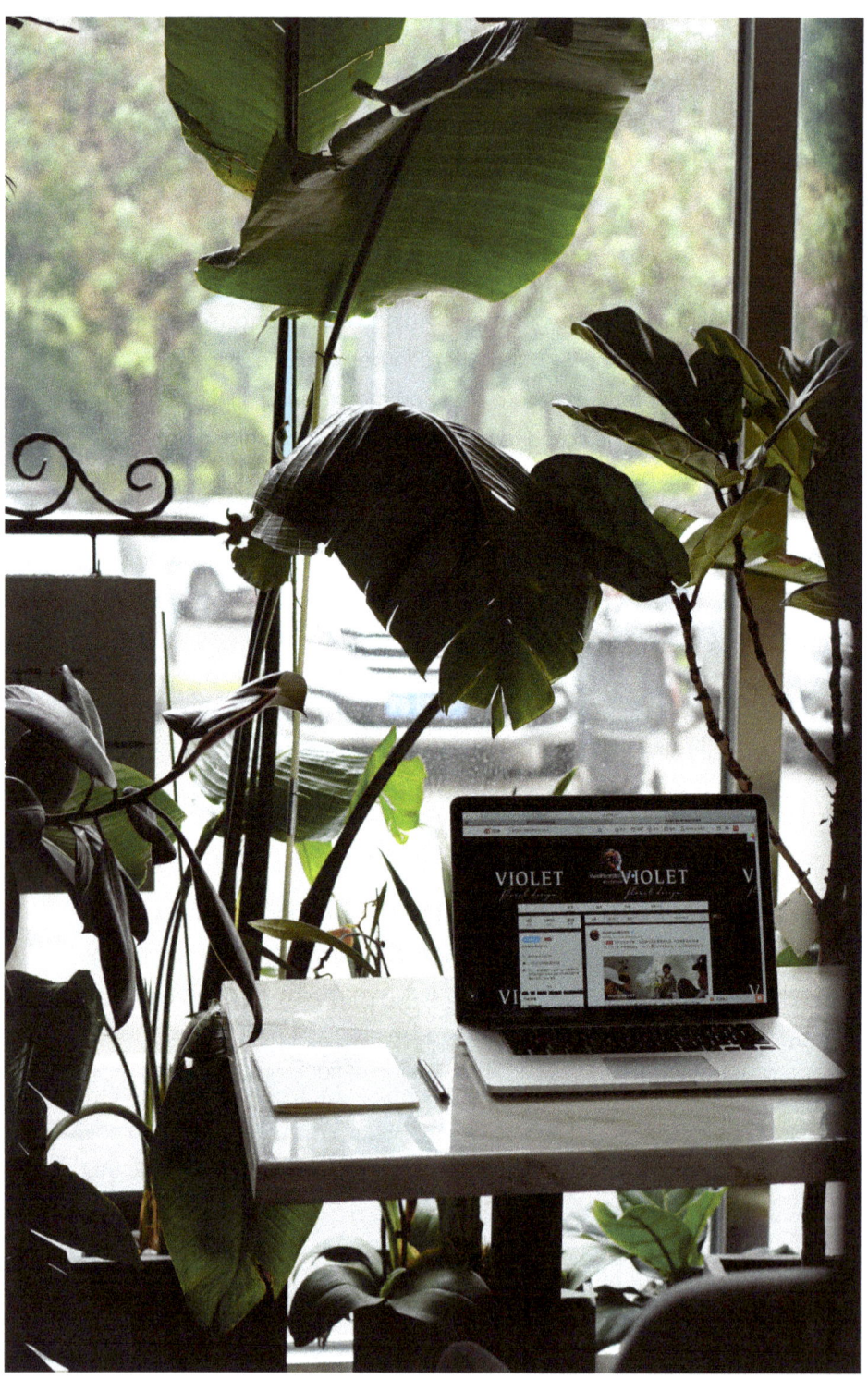

Section Four: Setting the Stage

At this point, you're probably done with hard decisions, emotional introspectives, and difficult conversations. I am happy to report that, for the most part, that particular inner turmoil is behind you. That doesn't mean every day will be fantastic, and that your job will be nothing but fun and productive. Instead, you are now equipped with a significant amount of information and a new understanding about yourself. Now it's time to do some prep work that requires less soul searching and more construction.

Now that you have been granted the opportunity to take your career out of the office- or made the tough decision to drop everything and start anew- you need to prepare for that actual transition. You've done the tough work in getting mentally organized for this change, so now let's get physically prepared!

Chapter One: Creating Your Work Space

Regardless of the job you plan to do, or whether you're planning on working from your home, a van, a skoolie, or a yurt, you're going to need to figure out the logistics of your work space.

At the bare minimum, you're going to need to find a spot where you can comfortably spread out all of your equipment and work materials, with adequate access to all of the resources you need to get you through your day. You may be thinking, "well, I did see that really cool desk at that antique store, so I think I'll get that." That's fine. Bookmark that. But before you start filling up your space with the things that inspire you, you have to *find* that space.

If you're planning on taking your job back to your home, you might think this is a super-easy decision. You'll turn the corner of the spare room into an office, or prop up a collapsible desk in front of the sofa, or maybe you'll just set up shop at the dining room table. Logically, all of these are fine ideas, depending on your available space. But will you actually want to work there?

When Brad first started working from home, he set up his office in an upstairs room we used for workout equipment. He chose this spot for several reasons:
- It was quiet and away from the rest of the flow of the house
- He could have his own room AND his own bathroom
- He could shut the door to keep out our dog (who loved to bark when anyone was on speakerphone)
- When he worked late, it didn't disrupt the things I needed to do

Logically sound, right? In fact, on paper, it couldn't be more ideal. Unfortunately, the reality was completely different.

It turns out that the top floor of the house didn't get the same amount of air circulation as the rest of the house. While the windows were situated at the east and west ends of the room, and let in a great deal of breeze, they also let in the sun all day long, baking Brad from sunrise to sunset. The ceiling of the room was also too low to install a fan, so the only option at the time was to run noisy floor fans that had to be turned off for conference calls and Skype meetings.

Adding to the noise was the fact that the windows looked directly over the street, so any ambient neighborhood sounds immediately made their way onto conference calls. That included our beagle scratching at the closed door any time he felt he should be included on those calls. What was an ideal space for our workout equipment was a terrible place to try to concentrate for 8-12 hours straight. It didn't take long for Brad to discover that working at the kitchen table was a far better option for him, though he did briefly experiment with our semi-finished basement and even the garage.

Working in the van, on the other hand, is an entirely different matter. Brad has a tote that he calls his "office." It includes a folding stool, his laptop case, all of his charging cords, a canopy that can be easily unfolded and set up, and a cushion for the stool. His "desk" is a foldable unit that's reminiscent of a card table and those metal tv trays my grandparents used to occasionally eat dinner in the living room.

Each day- weather willing- he sets up his "office" under the canopy, taking care to remain within the range of our WiFi signal. If the weather is poor, he either sets up his laptop on top of our storage units and works inside the van, or he'll head to town to find a location with free Wi-Fi until the weather breaks. One such location that is surprisingly perfect is the laundromat. He can take advantage of WiFi to work while simultaneously plowing through our endless stream of dirty laundry.

Then there are people like me. I work best when I change location several times throughout the day. I tend to lock into one spot, pound out a few thousand words, take a stretch break, find a spot that appeals to me more, then head to that spot for another few thousand words. While Brad thinks a stool is comfortable, my achy back and I disagree. I'll usually start out in the bed area of the van with an assortment of pillows. Then, as the inside of the van heats up under the sun, I'll take my folding chair and lap desk out to catch the breeze. If the weather isn't great, and we're not set up at the laundromat (or a cafe, restaurant, or on a few notable occasions, a brewery), I'm the type that will find every potential working position in that tiny space.

The idea of having a fixed office space makes me feel incredibly trapped and slightly claustrophobic, which you might find funny, considering I live in a van. But let's look at the difference between our jobs. Brad does a ton of objective problem solving. He needs quiet and concentration and the ability to focus on really big problems. On the completely opposite side of the career map, I'm creative. I need to keep myself inspired and focused. If I stare at the same thing too long, I get bored. When I get bored, my mind starts wandering. When my mind starts wandering, so do I, and pretty soon I'm chasing butterflies or Googling information none of my current clients care about, like the type of car Columbo drove, or the lyrics to a song I listened to in high school.

I share these examples to demonstrate that work space is not one-size-fits-all, and that you may have to try a few different things out before you find the area that works best for you. You may have additional variables in your equation, like pets or children who are bound to make noise and require attention. If you have a bad back, or history of carpal tunnel flare ups, ergonomics are definitely something to keep in mind, as well. Don't settle for just any spot because you like the view. Make sure it works from a 360-degree approach!

Therefore, my recommendation to you is to come up with a few options for your work space. As mentioned earlier, the only real requirement is that you have enough room to set up all of your equipment and have access to any connectivity that is required of your job.

Let's look at what you need to work, equipment-wise. For nearly everyone, that's going to include a laptop. Even if you plan on pursuing a creative side-hustle, you'll still need a way to market your product. You might also require a label printer to print off addresses and postage for shipping. You'll also need whatever supplies are required to make your amazing product, and a way to store those supplies, whether at home or on the road.

I recommend starting with a list of everything you need to get things moving. For me, that looks like this:

- Laptop
- Charging cord
- Cell phone
- Caffeinated beverage
- Headphones
- Pillow to prop up laptop on my actual lap
- Notebook with dividers and pen

As you can see, I've included everything I can think of that I'll need. This prevents me from doing the whole "Ooh. I need to go get..." distraction routine. If I have my set up all planned out, I am entirely ready to go for the day.

Once you've gathered everything you need, figure out how to make it fit. If you're a desk person, this is probably super easy. If you're working from home, it may take a little finessing. But if you're working on the road, you've got to figure out where to put your drink so it won't spill on something important, and the phone has to go somewhere it can't fall in between cracks or make its way under something. The charge cords have to reach the power center, and don't you dare wander too far away from the WiFi!

Before your first day of working away from the office, walk through this process. Figure out what works and what doesn't. I will say that the greatest detractor from productivity in a work from home scenario is finding your stuff. Even at home, Brad would set his phone down when getting a cup of coffee and then spend the next fifteen minutes searching for it. Factor in the small nooks and crannies of a van or skoolie, and you can understand why preparedness and organization are key!

While you're in the process of conducting this dry run or walk through, make it a point to actually boot up your equipment. Make sure you can actually connect to any services you need to connect to, such as WiFi or a phone signal. At our house in Ohio, it was impossible to get a consistent phone signal in the basement or the front bedroom, and the WiFi didn't work directly in front of the fireplace. If you haven't explored the possibilities, you may not be aware of these types of dead zones until you're on the clock, so take the time to check things out before you try to log on for your first official day.

Setting up your work space may be one of the most objectively simple tasks on your list, but that doesn't mean it will be effortless. Giving your work space some conscious thought and deliberate design will aid your daily productivity. You'll not only stay on track by having everything where it needs to be, but you won't be distracted by trying to make things "perfect" when something doesn't feel or work right. You know your workflow better than anyone, so make sure your space is adequate for getting the job done.

Chapter Two: Understanding How to Work in a New Place

How do you work? If you've worked in a separate location your entire career, you may say, "well, I go to my place of employment, I clock in, and I start working." And that's a great start! But that's all about to change.

Walk yourself through a typical day in the office. You walk in, sure. Do you go straight to your desk, or do you detour to get a coffee or maybe some breakfast on your way? Once you arrive at your desk or work station, what's the first thing you do? Do you take a few moments to get yourself organized for the day, or do you jump right in by checking email or voicemail while you're still taking off your jacket?

Whether we like it or not, humans are most productive when they adhere to a routine. That's not necessarily a hard-and-fast rule, but once you start to examine your current work patterns a bit more, you'll realize that you tend to do things similarly each day.

For example, I wake up, start the coffee, wash up, and do a little brisk walk/jog around our camping area to get the blood flowing. Then I open up my laptop and start getting things organized while I desperately chug my coffee, waiting for its eye-opening effects to kick in. Brad wakes up, grabs a cup of coffee in a to-go mug, and wanders around for a good half hour, stimulating his senses into waking up with a nice walk. He washes up on his way back to the van, then sets up his office, and dives right in. One of our van life friends has the most astounding pre-work ritual I've ever heard of. He hikes at least 5 miles, chugs a can of craft beer, makes breakfast, and is ready to go by 9am EST every single day. He owns his own marketing firm, and despite his odd routine, does quite well for himself.

On your first day working remotely, you may feel a bit lost and stranded, especially if you've never worked outside of the traditional office setting. You might feel equal parts anxious to get the day started and excited by the idea that you can sleep in a little bit, since you don't have to get dressed up or drive anywhere. You may have added some new duties, like getting the kids ready for school, walking the dog, or getting breakfast ready for your household.

Regardless, this is another part of the day where a quick run-through before this becomes your actual process is beneficial. You don't have to practice until you have it down perfectly, but for many of us, learning through experience can help us develop our stride.

Once you've considered the start to your day, the rest of the work day should unfold somewhat naturally… or will it? If you're the type of person who does very well working on your own, who can moderate mental breaks, distractions, and productivity without interacting with others, then yes, you should be as good as gold.

On the other hand, if you're the type of person who likes to visit with other coworkers, and often collaborates on projects with other people in your office, you might suddenly feel incredibly lonely. You won't have the opportunity to stand up and walk to someone else's desk to ask their opinion on a specific issue. Depending on the technology available, you can send them an instant message, email, or call them, but it's not going to be the same.

You may discover that your new work environment is oppressively quiet. If you're completely alone, you may feel a brand new sense of isolation and almost abandonment. The people who once shared almost all of your waking hours are now spending that time without you, while you are all alone. They're laughing and joking at impromptu breakroom meetings, going to lunch together, bringing in treats to share with the office, and you aren't taking part in any of that.

If you are a very collaborative, team-oriented type of person, you will find this newfound solitary environment more distracting than anything you could have possibly imagined. Your dog could actually begin singing- not just the songs of his people, but Ave Maria- and it wouldn't be nearly as confounding as this isolation.

Then again, you may be the type of person who enjoys micromanagement, and you feel most in control and confident when someone is dictating exactly what you should be doing at every given moment. Many people feel like a boat floating away from its mooring when they first start working remotely. If you're going from a very tight-knit environment with clear, constant direction to freelancing, you're going to feel a bit lost at first. Now, if you feel that you have "escaped" that type of scenario, where you found the expectations of coworkers and management unrealistic and oppressive, then you're in the right spot. But if you're the type who second-guesses yourself every time you hit the spacebar on your keyboard, the transition will seem strange.

One recommendation I have for those who are more collaborative, or require more direction, is to try very hard to maintain that same level of connection. That can mean setting up quick phone calls with people to check in, or having day-end meetings with your boss to check up on everything. You might even suggest a weekly video conference with your team so you can all touch base on what you've done for your respective projects.

If you're changing fields entirely, don't let that be a reason to give up your professional connections. Remember that list of contacts you made earlier? Touch base with them. Be honest with them, too. "I'm feeling a little lost about starting this 'running my own business' thing. Can we take some time to talk about your experiences when you first started running your own show?" Anyone who has made this type of transition will relate to the myriad of feelings you're having, ranging from freedom to fear and independence to isolation. You're not nearly as alone as you feel.

Not only is your work style going to change significantly, but your work environment, as well. Every office building has some level of ambient noise, due to various parties being on the phone, holding meetings, etc. All of the elevator dings, street noise, mechanical whirrs, and the hum of the HVAC become subtly embedded in your brain, and you learn to work in that type of environment.

So when you've been working for a few hours, and you don't hear the elevator or hear your children's morning cartoon instead of a dull murmur of productivity, you may feel a bit displaced.

Try experimenting with different ambient sounds. I mentioned earlier that I prefer binaural beats, because music with words distracts me. Brad prefers 1980s hair bands, because the beat is fast and furious. I wrote an entire textbook to "Star Trek: The Next Generation," because I wanted to emulate the tone of Captain Jean-Luc Picard. You have complete permission to create the brain space you need to work efficiently.

One particular peril of working on the run is that you don't really have control over your environment. Brad and I were thrilled to find that we had a campsite in Alabama all to ourselves (hooray for the off-season!), until the maintenance crew came in at 11am on the dot to start mowing, trimming branches, and making all kinds of ruckus. Some campsites are filled with children and dogs who will make lots of noise starting at exactly 7am every day… in fact, some of those children and dogs may be your own! You can't control what the people around you are doing, so this is a situation where you'll have to evaluate if you need to take things to town, or if you can work with the windows up and headphones on for a bit.

Learning how to work in an entirely different environment can present some unexpected challenges. We'll look into dealing with some of the emotional and psychological changes in the next section, as well. In the process of creating your physical work space, you can take charge of as many challenges as you can recognize before getting started. That includes finding the ideal desk/chair/room situation, figuring out your start of day flow, and understanding what type of worker you are so you can meet any distractions head-on.

Chapter Three: Time to Work!

The next challenge is creating your work schedule. This is particularly important for freelancers, side-hustlers, and van folks of all industries.

The temptation to slack off will be incredibly strong at first. The distractions will be off the charts. For those starting out with freelancing and side-hustle gigs, when clients and projects are at an all-time low, you may feel that this is the opportunity to do nothing. Granted, folks in this position do have a bit more freedom than others, but doing nothing all day, everyday isn't the best option.

Instead, everyone who is making this full-on transition needs to think about creating a schedule. This schedule must not only make sense with your lifestyle, but with the tasks you need to complete, too .

This whole process started with an awareness of changes you need to make in your lifestyle in order to truly live. Whether that means carving out time for appointments, working fewer hours, working in the middle of the night, or taking a great big break in the middle of the day, your schedule should reflect exactly what your mind and body need in order to survive and thrive. You should have time to eat, take care of your personal needs, and get a satisfactory amount of work completed each day.

You also need time to rest. That amount differs for all of us. Some people are mentally and physically equipped to go for days on end, then crash for a day, get up, and do it all over again. Others may need a cat nap during the day to recharge. Whatever your body needs, allow it. While taking a thirty minute snooze at your desk during lunch break might be frowned upon, getting thirty minutes of shut eye on your sofa after eating a sandwich is no big deal. No one will ever know! You have the control factor. You have the freedom. Do whatever it takes to help yourself flourish in this new situation.

Then there are the tasks you need to complete. The "work" part of every "work/life" balance must not be ignored. Starting a career in freelancing or performing a side-hustle is not unlike the experience of a freshman starting college. You get your assignment and the due date, but how you get there is up to you. You could study up on the topic rigorously, attending every possible lecture, taking copious notes, and adding a bit to your project each day. Or, you can devote that energy and ambition to whatever feels like fun, and cap it all off with a series of all-nighters right before the big due date.

In this metaphor, of course, there are no lectures to attend, but the concepts are pretty similar. If a client gives you a due date that's a month out, you can choose to start research and preparations now, or you can wait until the last minute. Maybe you work best under pressure and have chosen only projects that you can complete quickly. As long as you get that final project in on time, and the client loves it, you'll pass the metaphorical class.

There are plenty of exercises you can try out to help keep your head in the game. In speaking with others who have made the transition to working from home or on the road, I learned that sometimes you have to trick yourself into being more disciplined than you want to be. Here are some of the tricks I've compiled from my own experiences and conversations with others who have left the office behind:

1. **Give yourself tighter deadlines.** Even if the assignment isn't due for a week, get it done faster. That way, you don't have the ability to slack off and hate yourself for it.

2. **Make your breaks meaningful.** Absolutely get up and stretch and move every 30-60 minutes- but don't take this as an opportunity to find a new distraction. Don't turn on the TV, don't even think about logging on to social media, and definitely don't get yourself caught up in a personal project that's going to drag your mind away for hours. Take a brief, brisk walk. Have a snack. Doodle. Meditate. Do some yoga. Do anything that you can immediately drop after 10-15 minutes without effort.

3. **Plan out a rough schedule for your week.** I personally hate lists and schedules, because when things go sideways, I become a giant ball of anxiety and guilt. However, if you create even the most bare-bones outline of your day or week, it will help you know what you need to accomplish. You'll also be abundantly aware of deadlines that are creeping up on you.

4. **Stick to your schedule.** This is INCREDIBLY hard for freelancers and side-hustlers, because you may have a few days where you are not required to get up early and pound out a project. You want to sleep in, breathe deep, and just stare at the wall. That's completely valid, but once work picks up again, you'll feel bitter that you don't have the same amount of slack off time you had earlier. Give yourself time to rest and recover- especially after difficult projects- but keep your mind involved and active.

5. **Choose a hobby that has nothing to do with your occupation.** Since I've made reading and writing my job, I don't find sitting down with a good book as relaxing as it used to be. Instead, I fire up an audio book and listen to a fabulous tale while I draw or color. After a long day of looking at a computer screen, I absolutely adore setting up my yoga mat outside and following along with an online yoga flow. Brad is a runner, so the unspoken rule is that he will hang up the phone, close his laptop, deconstruct his office, lace up his shoes, and come back after a few miles of jogging it out. You need something to look forward to and a method that truly helps you re-engage with the life part of the work-life balance.

These are just a few tips from those of us who have been there and done that. You may accidentally discover a technique that really works for you. Enjoy the control you have earned by leaving the office environment, and do what makes you feel more productive and encourages you to keep working. Inspiration is literally everywhere. If the "Hang In There, Baby" poster from your desk space did something for you, hang it up in your workspace. Make it your laptop wallpaper. You no longer have coworkers to get irritated by it, so go ahead and click your pen endlessly for 45 minutes. Keep your brain focused in a way that's meaningful for you, and the productivity will follow!

Creating the perfect physical, mental, and emotional space for success in your new endeavor requires a little more effort than you might initially imagine. You may need to spend the first few months of your new work scenario figuring out exactly what works for you, and ironing out all the details. This may be frustrating, but ultimately, you will find your stride. Oftentimes, this happens quite organically, as you settle in with your new routine. Other times, you will have to experiment with ways to motivate yourself out of bed, and to coax yourself into sitting down and working, even when you really don't want to do a single thing. Personally, I would say it was about a year before I really felt like I was doing things "right" for me. You may need more or less time. Just know that no one has ever found this to be a quick and easy process, and you are truly never alone!

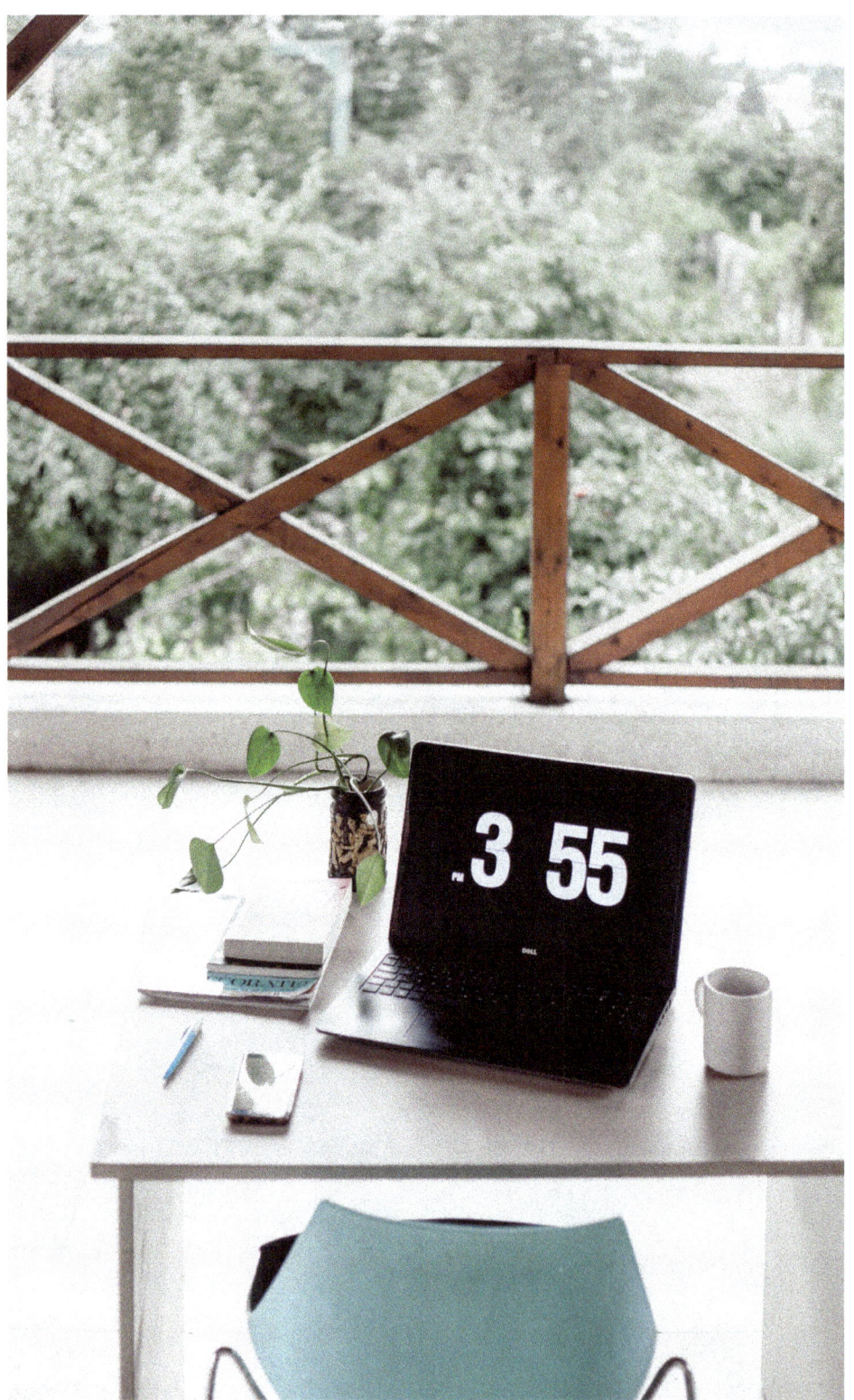

Section Four: Finding Your Stride and Making It Work

Now that you've got your plan in hand, it's time to make it work. Don't be surprised if you experience some growing pains along the way, however. You've just changed your entire working model, so there are a few aspects of your overall attitude, daily experience, and long-term success that might change radically. Still, it is possible to turn these growing pains into incredible experiences, so that you might be truly successful in a career that rewards you not just financially, but emotionally, as well.

Chapter One: The Social Aspect

Earlier, we touched on how your work environment will drastically change your interactions with others. Many of us thrive in an office environment due to the social aspect, either because of the opportunities for collaboration and direction, or through commiserating with our fellow employees. We make friends in the office, some of whom become very near and dear to us. The concept of an "office spouse" or "office bestie" is not unheard of, because many of us gain very close relationships with those who understand and appreciate exactly what we go through for the majority of our waking hours.

Once you take yourself out of that environment of closeness and camaraderie, you may feel a deep sense of isolation. This is perfectly natural. For those who are simply transitioning the same job they've had in the past to a home office, it's a great idea to continue to meet up with coworkers for lunch or happy hours, so that you can retain that social connection.

But what if you're changing jobs completely? If you're permanently leaving the office behind for a freelance lifestyle or the ultimate side-hustle, you may feel like you're saying goodbye. It's true that some things about your friendship will change. You won't be at the same level for venting sessions or office chatter, but you don't have to walk away from a beautiful bond just because the situation has changed. Meet up for coffee, connect via social media, and invite each other to social gatherings. You may be surprised to discover that your former coworkers will simply love seeing you at the occasional happy hour, and they'll have tons of questions about your new gig- along with a little residual jealousy.

Van life folks have it the hardest when it comes to the changes in the social aspect of working on the run. You are voluntarily stuck in a small, enclosed vehicle, all day, every day, with the same person. Granted, the opportunity for isolation exists, as demonstrated by Brad taking off with his office-in-a-tote while I occupy the van, but the only people you have to complain/vent/exalt to regularly are those who are also seated in the same vehicle.

At first, they'll be fascinated with your stories, especially if you are both new to this job or environment. You'll excitedly chatter over an evening meal, relishing that pre-bedtime glass of wine or mug of cocoa as you rehash the day to mentally process everything that has happened. Eventually, you will reach what I call the "Who Cares?" phase, in which one person speaks while anyone else present rapidly forgets how to listen. This stage can be difficult, because it's fairly easy to tell when no one is paying attention to you. Over time, this morphs into a sense of personal involvement, when you realize you've become deeply entrenched in each other's work, despite having only the faintest clue of what they're doing and how it happens. You may find yourself coming up with nicknames for people you've never met, and starting sentences with "you should tell them... ." It may not be healthy, but it's a very real step in the bonding process of people who work in solitude.

In the office, Brad was "kind of a big deal." He had people stopping at his desk from the moment he walked in the door until the automatic timers shut off the lights for the evening. He was invited to nearly every team's social functions, both work related and personal.

When he started working from home, a lot of that stopped. Not only did he lose the constant stream of visitors, but the invites started trailing off, as people who would extend those invitations in elevators, breakrooms, and the parking garage lost sight of him. Though he's not an extrovert by any means, losing the social aspect was pretty depressing. He felt an extreme sense of isolation. Thankfully, he adapted by the time he started working on the road, but it was a lengthy period of coping.

For me, the sense of loneliness hit almost immediately after we pulled out of the driveway. I'm also an introvert, but I rely heavily on my network for regular interaction and connection. I was used to seeing the same coworkers each day, laughing, complaining, crying, and sharing snacks with them. Being on the road took all of that away from me. In fact, I stopped having my 3pm snack altogether! While that was a great move for weight loss, the sense of losing my group was painful.

There are a few things you can do to ease this transition into solitude. A few of the methods we used include:

1. **Find your favorite noise.** I've mentioned music, podcasts, and audio books a few times. These are actually great ways to make your brain feel less lonely. You get to hear sounds and voices and get information, even when no one is around. One method I enjoy is putting a documentary on for background noise while I make meals. I love information. I love hearing other humans' voices. I can learn all about British castles while making dinner, and while the host will never hear my witty commentary, I get to hear his charming remarks.

2. **Stay connected.** Your network is key. Text your friends and family. Keep up with your social media. Heck, if the phone connection is strong enough, call them! One fun activity that helped get me through the first year of van travel was sending postcards to a friend. The messages started out short enough- after all, there's very little room on a postcard. Soon, I was explaining why the postcard made me think of her, and the story of how that postcard ended up in the mail to her. Plus, finding stamps and post boxes is a challenge in itself that can keep you occupied for hours (for extra fun, don't use a GPS)!

3. **Talk to strangers.** If reading that sentence makes you feel queasy and uneasy, you're not alone. The first few months of van living found me fully tongue tied. I felt uneasy speaking to anyone, because I was truly a "stranger in a strange land." I didn't know anyone, and I didn't belong. It wasn't until Brad ended up fielding a work call at a brewery in Montana that I suddenly felt a pressing need to make new friends. Perhaps the strong brew eased my apprehension, but soon I was chatting about van life with the woman sitting next to me, the bartender, and two little boys who came in with their father.

    Not everyone is receptive to meeting new people, and I'm certainly not saying you should put yourself on the threshold of danger. But being out and about, sharing a few friendly words with fellow hikers, folks at restaurants and cafes, neighbors at camping spots, and more can be soothing to the soul. It can also be highly productive, as your interaction may reveal some cool ideas for things to do, restaurants to try, and fantastic views. A chance interaction with a fellow in a restaurant in Idaho led to a quickly sketched map to a free camp spot in the National Forests. From there, Brad and I were treated to the most stunning sunset we have ever experienced. It can truly pay off to learn from the locals through casual conversation.

4. **Find events to attend.** From car rallies to county fairs, there is always something happening, somewhere. You can find inexpensive and free events to pop into briefly until your social craving is whetted. If you find that you're enjoying yourself, stay a spell. Brad and I have done all sorts of things that we wouldn't have done at home, from going to a rodeo, to attending a lecture on the socio-psychological turmoil experienced by those involved in the Western Expansion. We've appeared at art gallery events, beer releases, and even a book release for a tome about Sasquatch. If you need a crowd, it's easy to find one. Plus, these experiences become some of the highlights of your van life adventure.

I won't say it's easy to move forward, and I certainly can't say that this feeling of solitude will go away. Even if it's the thing that most excited you about van life during the planning stages, you'll have a certain feeling of disconnection as you physically distance yourself from the world you once knew. You don't have to give up your friendships, however. You just need to learn how to help them evolve.

Chapter Two: The Growth Aspect

"Where do you see yourself in ten years?" Anyone who has been to a job interview, performance review, or motivational career event has heard that question. And despite the fact that we fumble through a few words about growth, success, and learning, the truth is, we often have no idea. Personally, I can't picture dinner when I wake up in the morning. How am I supposed to know what my life is going to look like in a decade? I don't know what the economy will look like, or what marketing trends will be, and I don't know if the van is going to last another ten years, and... there are a lot of "what ifs" on everyone's horizon.

One area in which you have control is your career. You have already demonstrated that when you made the decision to leave the traditional office setup. And while that's probably plenty to deal with for now, eventually you will want to progress somehow.

Whether you're maintaining your current role or planning on knitting scarves from the back of a van, your career is not immune to growth. Maybe you're small bananas now, but every job, craft, art, occupation, past-time, and opportunity has the ability to lead you somewhere on your life's path.

When I started freelancing, some of my first gigs were writing 300-word "About" pages for $5 a pop. They required about thirty minutes of research and ten minutes of writing. But I took as many as I could handle, and I wrote my heart out. Now I'm reading, editing, and writing books full time. Who knows where I'll be in a year, two years, or more?

Maybe you're happy knitting scarves in the back of your van. That is completely respectable. I love handmade items, and scarves are a great source of warmth for people who don't have central heat or think that ice hiking is fun. But maybe, as the slips and purls go by, you're thinking about how you can combine your knitting skills with your motivational skills, and create an opportunity in which your scarf sales can benefit others. Maybe you're planning a non-profit in which your scarves can be donated to the homeless, and create a mission from there. No job is small. No creation is without impact.

If growth is something you crave, I encourage you to pursue it. How? There are several ways:

- **Learn.** Distance learning is easier now than it ever has been, with online programs that can help you advance your knowledge in marketing yourself and your skills. If you find a weak spot that is preventing you from getting to where you dream of being, apply your energy towards learning more. Do the research. Take the courses. Listen to the lectures.
- **Network**. I've said it before: you are not alone. Find the community, and become part of the niche. Look for mentors and companions on this journey. If Frodo could convince Samwise to walk with him to Mordor, then surely you can find others who can get on board with your fantastic idea.
- **Stay connected**. Or rather, don't be oblivious. When I started writing, I had no idea that MLA-style was no longer a thing. All of the lessons I'd been taught, all of the terrible marks I'd received for grammatical errors were no longer valid. In this day and age, a lot of the rules have changed. For example, it's ok to start sentences with the word "However." If I had a time machine, I'd love to go back to college and apprise a few professors of these facts, but unfortunately, that technology doesn't exist. What this means is that when I started freelancing, I received a whole bunch of comments on my outdated style. That's entirely my fault- I didn't stay connected to learn about these changes. You'll have far better success with growth if you keep your finger on the pulse of your industry.

- **Be honest about it**. Tell your boss, your clients, and your network of your personal aspirations. You can't make your dreams a reality if you pretend they don't exist. If you explain to your boss that you'd like to make your way to Director level in the next three years, chances are very good that they'll be able to provide you with tips and goals that will take you down that path. If you're performing well for a client in a freelance scenario, and you mention that you're looking for something more, they may very well be happy to accommodate that growth with additional projects and increased responsibility.

But what if, in the lexicon of our youth, you "don't wanna?" You have control now. You don't have to grow. You don't have to aspire to take over a Fortune 500 company by the time you're fifty- unless you want to. You can write the Great American Novel, or you can cheerfully write web content and product descriptions for the rest of your working life. You can start a world-wide charity based on your scarf knitting, or you can do nothing more wild than finishing a sweater. It's all up to you.

In the office environment, I found that the need to rise up the proverbial ladder, to smash the glass ceiling and rule the world, and to continuously have motion within the corporate hierarchy was more of an expectation than my own personal desire. Sure, everyone loves an increase in pay, but the drastic increase in responsibilities that come with that bigger check sometimes outweighs the benefits.

When you first started to consider working remotely, as we did in the first chapter, you came to realize that the picture is a little bigger than your specific role within the org chart. This is especially true if your reasons for leaving the office are for family or personal issues. As that disconnect from the social aspect kicks in, you might start to feel like you'll never advance in your career, but that's simply not true. Compromising personal needs and your career should always work out in your favor.

A wise mentor of mine once told me, "for me, it's more important to become valuable for what I do, not how much of it I do." That is to say, prioritize your own well-being, enjoy your lifestyle, and don't burn out.

Chapter Three: The Financial Aspect

Maybe I've read too many "how to" financial advice books (ironically, for a client), but one question that will always intrigue me is the value of a dollar.

We tend to think about the financial aspect of our career in terms of amounts. When given a task to perform for pay, we see dollar signs, coin heaps and bills paid instead of hours spent, emotions invested, and brain power taxed. Somehow, the promise of financial gain makes us forget that work is hard.

Also, we obviously need money to live. I'd love to write a book called "How to Quit Your Job and Have Fun Doing Whatever You Want," but that's not in the cards right now. While working from home will help you save the money you would have spent on commuting, work clothes, and treating yourself to lunch or coffee every day, there are always expenses to count on. We all need food and shelter. Some of us need to put gasoline in our shelters every few hundred miles!

What I'm asking you to consider through all of this is the balance you want to make between the effort you make and the payment you take. This is true for anyone with a paying job, but there tends to be this wild misconception that anyone who isn't in the office magically has more time than anyone else. You may feel pressured to take on more tasks to "prove" that you can work from a remote location and still be productive, or you may find people wordlessly assigning you more projects.

For freelancers and side-hustlers, this is also very true, especially in the first few years. The first few years are stressful not just because you're trying to establish yourself, but because your brain and your body are not trained for this sudden change. The gig you choose may require more physical activity, and it will definitely engage new areas of your brain.

Even though I was an English major in college, where reading, researching, and reporting massive quantities of facts and ideas was something I did multiple times a day, that part of my brain had only been moderately simmering while I was working in a corporate human resources environment. When I first began writing full time, I found myself absolutely exhausted to the point where my computer screen would turn to gibberish after a few hours. My brain was just over tired.

You will likely approach your freelancing gigs and side-hustle activities with a violent fervor at first, and that energy is absolutely wonderful. Just make sure that you aren't putting in more effort than you're being compensated for.

At the same time, you need to balance cost of living with your income. For those remaining in their stationary homes, you'll already be aware of your general living expenses. But keep in mind that working from home means you don't have to live within a reasonable commute to the office. Depending on whether you still have to (or wish to) make in-person appearances, you now have the ability to take control over that part of your life, too. Once that twice-a-day commute is taken out of the daily equation, many people feel they have the freedom to work from areas where the cost of living is not quite as steep as it may have been otherwise.

For those transitioning to van life, your expenses are going to be very different. How different, or in what ways, depends on what type of vehicle you have, what type of adventure you've planned, and many other factors that I covered in "How to Live the Dream: Things Every Van Lifer Needs to Know." Whether you choose the gig first or the van life first, you will need to eventually align your expenses and income.

This may require a bit of experimentation, especially if you are new to both van living and freelancing or your side-hustle. Don't become discouraged, even though it can be very tempting to just give up. You can always go back to the drawing board and reconsider your options. That's the beauty of working for yourself: you can "quit" one job and take up another with just a few clicks of the mouse and an ounce of resolution.

In fact, I found myself re-evaluating my life choices about every month the first year. I'm lucky, in that Brad's steady income was present, and we had purposefully saved for our van life for a few years before we hit the road. But if I came to the end of the month and realized that I was quickly burning out, then noticed that I'd only made $100 in the entire month, that meant I wasn't doing it right. There will always be months that are sparse, unless you have regular clients. You can choose to respond by picking up more clients or gigs, or adding something else to your repertoire. Alternately, you can find a home base and "sit out" for a while to give your brain the option to come up with another plan!

Chapter Four: The Fear Aspect
One of the most common excuses that we tell ourselves is that "the time isn't right." This may seem especially resonant when you factor in the previously mentioned facts that you will be alone, that your career path may change, and that your financial situation will require a different level of attention than it has in the past.

When you start to have these sneaking feelings that maybe "the time isn't right," ask yourself if that's really the case, or if that's just the fear speaking. Both are extremely valid options, depending on your situation.

Let's look at a few ways that fear might be manifesting in your plans, and think of some questions to ask yourself to suss out whether it's real or anxiety:

Your Brain Says	Is It Real?	Is It Fear?
"If you leave now, you'll be passed over for that promotion."	• Does your employer have a history of giving remote workers the cold shoulder? • Do you have a history of shaky performance? • Are you really fully invested in receiving that promotion? Is it one of your Top 5 Goals at this moment?	• What is the worst thing that will happen if you do not receive this promotion? • Will receiving this promotion mean that you can't work from home or on the road? • If you wait until you receive the promotion to change your work situation, what other details of your life will also be put on hold?
"Things are just really busy right now, and transitioning out of the office would disrupt everything."	• Would the majority of your current job duties be impossible to perform from another location? • Is there no one else who can perform the tasks you regularly handle? • Is the success of this particular project or period in the office currently weighing on your mind more than the lifestyle you wish to pursue?	• Are you the most important cog in this particular wheel? • What would happen if a dire emergency kept you away from the office for an extended period of time? Would this task plunge into chaos? • When this task is complete, will you be ready to leave the office behind?
"I've only been in this job for a year. What will it look like if I leave now?"	• Is this a career path that you intend to follow for a significant period of time? • Is this particular job an incredibly valuable stepping stone to your overall life goals? • Will staying in this job provide you with opportunities you can't get anywhere else?	• Are you intimidated by the idea of having a frank discussion about altering your job situation with your management team? • Does the concept of failing at your attempt to work from the road or from home make you feel more uncomfortable than the idea of maintaining the status quo? • What factors in the first exercise led you to believe that working remotely was the best decision in the first place?

Ultimately, the question you need to ask yourself is, "Is it really better to wait?"

Sometimes, the answer is yes. You may not have the vehicle you need sitting in your driveway. You may have only $4 in your bank account until next Friday. You may have children who are attending school, family members who rely on you being exactly where you are now, or any of a variety of factors that make staying exactly where you are the right decision, right now.

That doesn't mean you can't start planning your exit strategy now. In fact, you have an advantage that many of us didn't necessarily consider when leaving the office behind. Nearly everyone has fantasized about walking into the boss's office on a particularly rough day, launching into a poignant rage-fueled (yet well-worded) speech about where anyone listening can put this job, grabbing the best chotchkies from their cubicle, and slamming the door behind them as they leave with a flourish.

You may be incredibly frustrated and confused and angry with the way things are going now. Or maybe you felt that way when you completed the exercises in Section One, but as you cool off, you realize there are a lot more moving parts than you originally considered. Maybe working remotely will eventually be the correct answer, but setting off at dawn tomorrow isn't the best option. That doesn't mean you have to officially close the book on this option. Instead, brainstorm the pieces that need to move- and where they need to go- so you can one day get to the job situation you crave.

I recommend anyone who is still wavering on whether the time is right take this short quiz:

1. Which is more important to you:
    a. Gaining wealth
    b. Earning higher status
    c. Living the best possible life

2. How far away is retirement for you? If you wait until then to pursue all of the things you're putting off by not working from home or the road, will you be:
   a. Perfectly happy
   b. Bitter and resentful
   c. Oh, I'm definitely not waiting that long. I'm a year out at max.

3. What is the number one thing that you need to make you feel comfortable with leaving the office?
   a. The moral support of friends, family, and coworkers
   b. Money
   c. A box to carry my stuff

4. Essay Question: What other changes have you put on hold because you're afraid?

There are no right or wrong answers to this quiz, of course. The intention is to get your brain moving. You can actually revisit these four questions any time you need to in the course of your life, to help think through any major decision.

For me, the urge to keep climbing the corporate ladder fizzled out when my division was sold. I was only 30, which meant I had 35 years of struggle ahead of me before I could retire– if I was lucky. Brad, on the other hand, made the decision that he wanted to retire at age 50, so he and his financial planner had been working on that model since his early twenties. I was not (and still am not) that level of a planner, so while I had all the retirement accounts set up, I'd never really thought about them. Wealth was obviously not a motivating factor for me. I was sick of the stress of an office job and a routine, so I would've answered "c" to the first question, and "b" to the second.

As for the other changes I put on hold due to fear? Too many to list! I am a very anxious person by nature, raised by two highly risk-averse individuals, married to someone who is sensible enough to have started investing at age 20. I am very good at being too afraid to change anything. In fact, I've had anxiety about wearing a different pair of socks while hiking, because the last time I changed my socks, something bad happened.

But that question- "is it really better to wait?"- kept haunting me.

At the end of the day, you are the only person in the entire world who can answer that question. There are compelling reasons on all sides of the argument, and there may be times when it is legitimately best to wait a bit. I suggest you make a list to help you figure out the pros and cons and any other angles that might appear. I recommend keeping a running list of thoughts over a period of time- perhaps a week, minimum.

In my case, I was definitely emotionally and physically prepared to leave the office behind, but not at all aware of the challenges that awaited me by starting a new career, working for myself, by myself, in a tiny blue van. Brad walked away from his desk with the three framed pictures he'd brought in and a heart full of ambition. His surprise came when the emotional and psychological aspects of being alone demonstrated that he was virtually "stranded" in his chosen work environment.

One or all of these intimidating concepts will arise over the next few years, perhaps together or individually. You may worry about being alone. You may become concerned that you'll do the same crummy task over and over for the rest of your life. Living from payment to payment may be a very real experience. You will frequently wonder if you have done the right thing.

But at the end of the day, will you regret it? I can't tell you the answer to that question, but for what it's worth, I haven't encountered anyone yet who does!

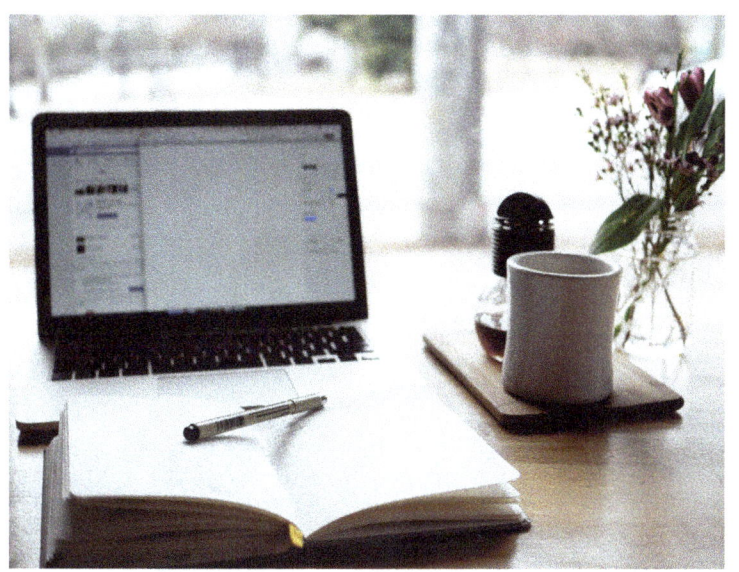

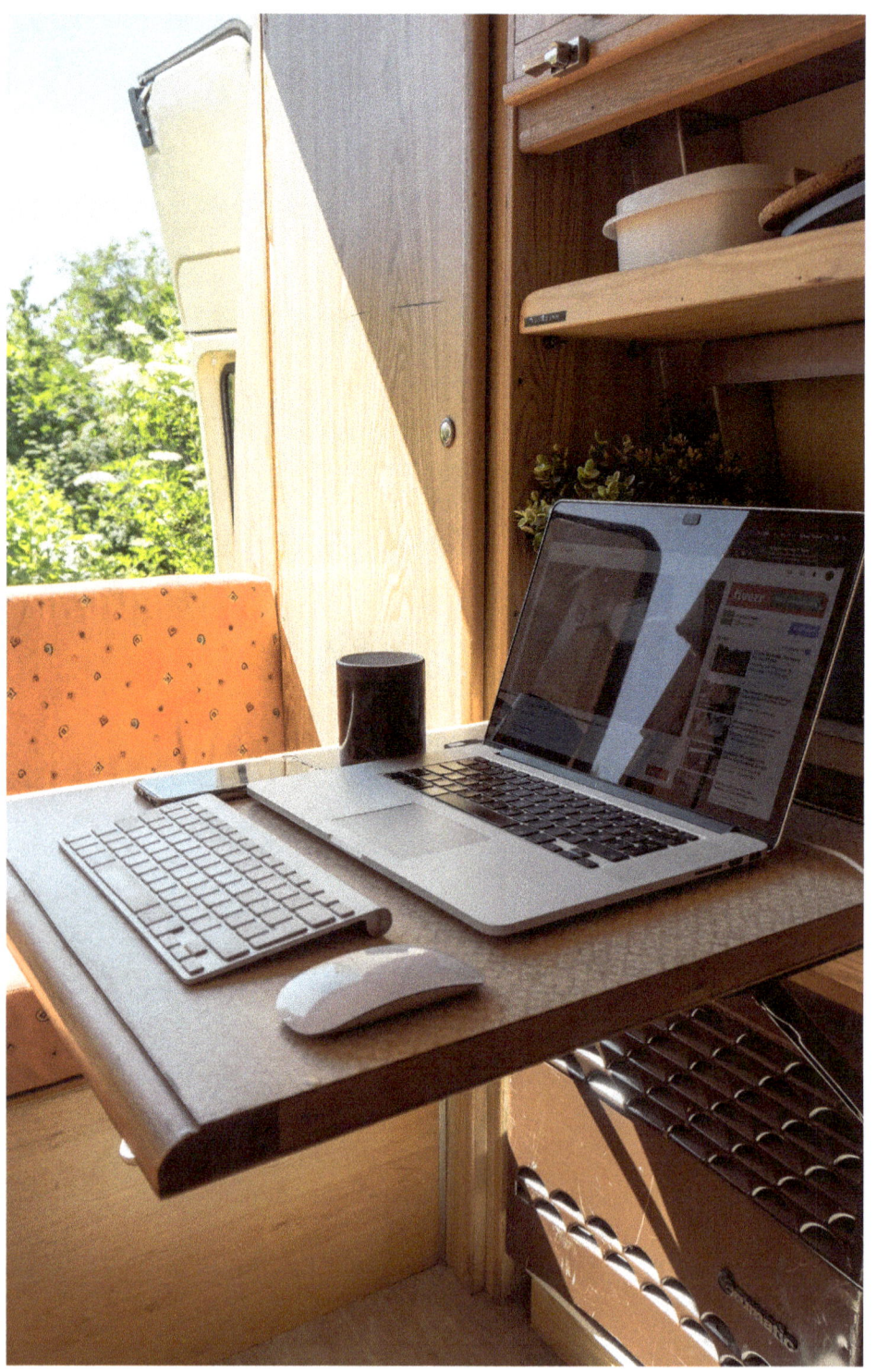

Section Five: Wrapping It All Up

I would love to be able to end this book by telling you that if you follow these tips, you'll be a millionaire, living your best life in the near future. But that's just not realistic for all of us.

My goal with the various exercises presented throughout this book was to help you get into the right mindset for taking your profession out of the office and into your own life. Thanks to technological advances and the connectivity provided by the internet, the possibilities today are far greater than they were just ten years ago. Corporate workers can attend meetings virtually. Freelancers can connect with an infinite number of clients located all over the world. Side-hustlers and crafters can advertise their wares to the entire planet by creating a simple website. Even day-by-day workers can find employment in the next town they plan to visit by conducting a quick search on their phones.

Finding a gig via the internet may be easier than ever, but maintaining that employment through all of life's changes can be difficult. No matter what type of occupation you pursue, your own personal situation will find a way to interrupt. In some cases, that's a temporary blip that can be accommodated by minor adjustments in your current career situation. In other cases, that interruption will lead to the discovery of a brand new lifestyle!

If I had been told at the start of my professional life- fresh out of college in 2002- that in a matter of years I'd be writing books in the back of a van, I probably would have believed it, but assumed the worst. Chris Farley's "Saturday Night Live" motivational speaker character, Matt Foley, cautioned my generation time and time again about the perils of "living in a van down by the river." I probably would have interpreted that fate as a warning, rather than the extremely positive, fulfilling scenario that plays out my life.

And yet, here I am, lucky enough to do my two most favorite things every single day: explore and write. I'll be the first to admit that it hasn't been smooth sailing the whole time. The van breaks down from time to time. I have had several dozen panic attacks accompanied by unseemly banshee-level shrieking when the WiFi connection disappears right before a major deadline. On one particularly quaint occasion, the van broke down, the generator stopped, and the water line broke. We were able to get out of that mess within a few hours thanks to some very kind fellow boondockers, but the life lesson learned from that is that the worst case scenario is not just possible, it's plausible!

I hope to leave you feeling well-prepared and encouraged about the transition to working remotely. There is never a wrong time to do the exercises recommended. My experience in corporate human resources has demonstrated the value of revisiting these types of questions from time to time.

The days of stagnating in the same job for 30 continuous years have passed. While it's certainly admirable, we now live in a world of opportunity and development. Whether you choose to grow in your current role, or try different things for the rest of your life, "variety" and "flexibility" are now two of the most treasured qualities in an employee.

This may not be the last time you consider your job and think, "am I really doing the right thing? Am I happy here?" I encourage you to think of this transition not as a final place to rest, but another step towards the next big change, all of which are set along the path towards living your best possible life.

For your convenience, I have rounded up the main questions asked throughout this text, so you can refer to them whenever you like. You might want to hang this list up in a conspicuous place, or use it as journalling fodder. However you get to these answers is perfectly fine, as long as you're honest with yourself!

Why do I want to work remotely?

How did I come to this potential decision?

What are some things I want to control?

What are some areas where I need more flexibility?

What are the pros and cons of working remotely?

What will I accomplish with this change?

Am I willing/able to take my current job on the road?

Am I interested in changing my career?

What are my talents, interests, and strong skills?

In my wildest dreams, what does my work/life balance look like?

How do I think this is going to work?

Who can I count on in my network?

How will I create my work space?

Do I have access to everything I need to get the job done?

What kind of schedule will work best for both my work and my lifestyle?

How do I inspire my own productivity?

What types of distractions might I encounter?

How do I work?

How important is the social aspect of your current work environment?

Where do you see yourself in ten years?

Do your expenses and income line up adequately?

Is it better to wait?

This is likely to be a very exciting and nerve wrecking time for you. You will likely experience many emotions and have many thoughts racing through your head. You might lose sleep as you try to organize your thoughts. There will be anxiety at the great unknown that lies ahead, but also great relief as you manage to capture more and more control over your work/life balance.

For everyone reading this, I wish you a smooth transition. I urge you to stay confident even when you're completely broken down on a Colorado mountainside. I strongly believe that our experiences shape us, and that what we consider "failure" is just another type of experience telling us we were heading down the wrong path.

To aid you on your quest, I've included a section of resources that I have found helpful and that have been recommended to me by others who have left the office to seek a greater purpose.

Read on, and may you find the footholds that you need to reach greatness!

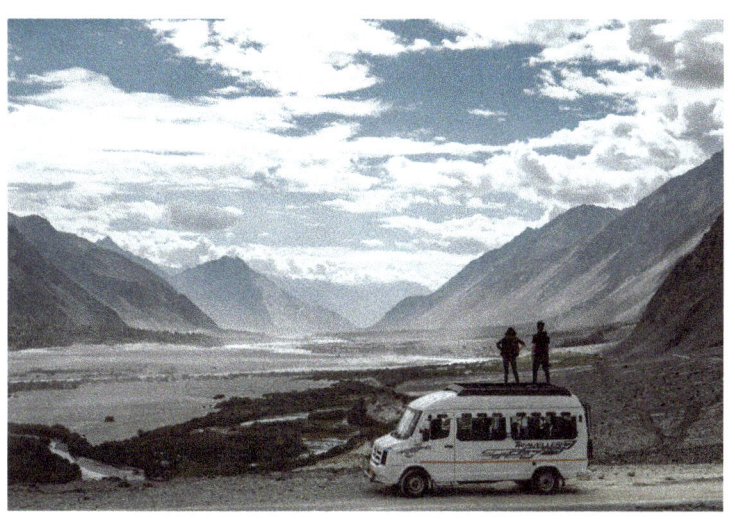

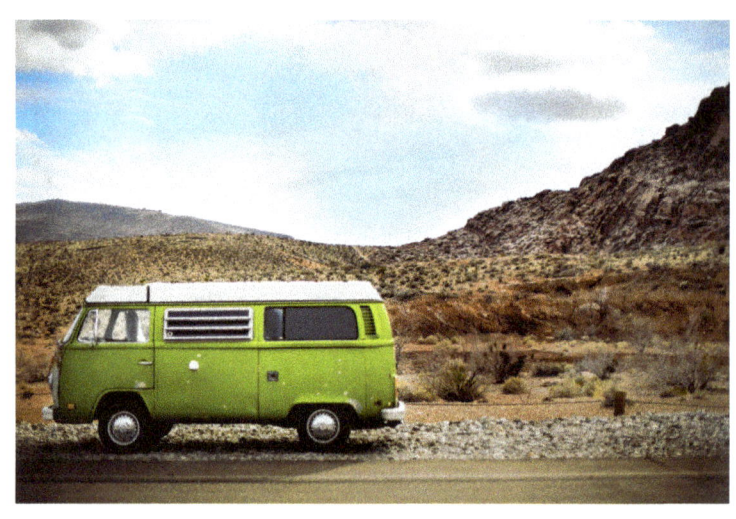

Section 6: Resources for Former Office Workers

I've included a few links to sites that could potentially help you find the direction you'd like to go in creating the ultimate work location and situation for yourself. There also are links to groups and organizations that should provide support with the potential challenges mentioned earlier, including the social, financial, productivity-vs-distractions aspects, as well as tips to create a practical physical and emotional space for your new work environment.

None of these links are intended to be considered endorsements, and may not reflect the opinions of those affiliated with this book. These sites were cultivated merely for the possible assistance they can provide to those who are looking to make huge maneuvers in their professional lives. This list is not exhaustive, either- instead, think of it as a launching pad for the things you wish to learn about in greater detail!

Productivity Management Resources

As mentioned several times, a change in work environment can impact your productivity. If you're the type who needs direct guidance to stay on task, or wouldn't mind a frequent reminder of due dates, appointments, and more, consider adding one of these resources to your daily structure.

My Life Organized: https://www.mylifeorganized.net/
Available for: iOS and Android, Windows
What it does: If you're the type of person who craves micromanagement, and whose "To Do" list looks more like the outline for a scholarly research paper, you might be the type to appreciate My Life Organized. This app breaks down all of your duties into tasks, all of your tasks into sub-tasks, and all of your lists into errands.

RescueTime: https://www.rescuetime.com/
Available for: iOS and Android
What it does: This app can be considered a Time Management or Productivity assistant, but really, it's an internet babysitter. RescueTime works in the background, keeping track of your internet behavior. If you're the

type who easily falls down internet rabbit holes, this is a way to keep you focused on your new goals, rather than getting distracted.

Timely: https://memory.ai/timely
Available for: iOS and Android, Mac and Windows
What it does: Timely is an AI app that pays attention to what you're doing so that it can learn how to be your ultimate productivity manager. It keeps track of your behaviors and tasks and creates schedules to help optimize your time. If you need help with accountability and staying on track with multiple projects, this type of AI app can be of assistance.

Toggl: https://toggl.com/
Available for: iOS, Mac, Android
What it does: Toggl is a time-tracking app that helps you see where you're spending the most of your time. It provides weekly, monthly, or annual reports to help you refocus on your time and efforts. This is helpful for anyone who wanders off chasing butterflies a bit too often!

Trello: https://trello.com/
Available for: iOS and Android, Mac and Windows
What it does: Trello is a visuals-based project management program. Think Pinterest, but instead of losing valuable hours adding things to your board, it helps you create a visual display of what you need to accomplish. This can help you maximize your efforts without added stress.

Money Management Resources
Whether you're making the full plunge to a new career or side-hustle, or you just want to stay on top with the changes that occur when you lose the long commute and wardrobe budget, these resources can help. The financial aspect of any change is something that truly has an impact on our lifestyles, whether we like it or not. If you're like me and struggle with anything more than basic math, consider a money management resource to keep you organized and apprised of your finances. Again, I'm not affiliated with any of these, but share them as popular options that exist.

Mint: https://www.mint.com/
Mint helps you keep track of all of your bills, all of your balances, and even your credit score from one central location. If you have memories of your parents spreading all of the bills, bank statements, and checks across the kitchen table once a month, consider all of that, only on one simple screen.

The Penny Hoarder: https://www.thepennyhoarder.com/
If you have a question that even potentially might impact your pocketbook, The Penny Hoarder probably has a few articles that can provide advice and guidance, covering a wide variety of topics that can help you understand where your money comes from and where it goes.

The Simple Dollar: https://www.thesimpledollar.com/blog-overview/
The key word in the title is "Simple." This blog is highly educational, especially for those who are taking control of their money in a new way. From scouting the best insurance products, to helping you understand how you can make your savings work for you, this blog covers it all.

Stacking Benjamins: https://www.stackingbenjamins.com/about/
This is a podcast, but a valuable resource. Whether you tune in while you drive your van into the sunset, or in your headphones during a break, there's a wide variety of very relatable financial discussions for nearly every person's situation

Wally: https://www.wally.me/
Wally is for visual learners. It provides users with options to track expenses, create and maintain a budget, organizes receipts and other financial documents, and can even help synchronize family expenses and earnings.

Technical Resources

I've divided this section up into "Home Office" and "Working on the Run," because while there is some overlap between the two scenarios, you likely won't have any trouble with WiFi installation in a home that doesn't have wheels and a motor. These resources range from workspaces to wires, and help with a lot of the "where" and "how can I" questions that might arise when setting up your new workspace.

For those who will be working from an office that doesn't move, here are a few helpful links:

Decor and Space Tips:
https://www.thespruce.com/how-to-set-up-a-workable-home-office-1977403
https://www.hgtv.com/design/rooms/other-rooms/10-tips-for-designing-your-home-office
Both The Spruce and HGTV.com are absolute rabbit holes of gorgeous design ideas and amazing aesthetics, but these practical articles are a good place to get started if you're not sure how to proceed.

Ergonomics:
https://www.mayoclinic.org/healthy-lifestyle/adult-health/in-depth/office-ergonomics/art-20046169
https://ergo-plus.com/workplace-ergonomics/
You may not realize it right now, but your office set up, including your desk, chair, keyboard, mousepad, and monitor are all set up to help you avoid long and short term pain. Your transition to a new work space should not need to coincide with an increase in chiropractic and massage expenses. Check out these tips to ensure you're in the best form possible.

For Those Working For Themselves:
https://www.thebalancesmb.com/setting-up-home-office-845850
The Balance Small Business has plenty of tips for new freelancers, side-hustlers, and small business owners. This particular article includes some interesting tips for creating a workspace… which you can then follow to other tips you might need.

For Parents:
https://hbr.org/2017/03/balancing-parenting-and-work-stress-a-guide

https://www.parents.com/parenting/work/life-balance/
https://www.forbes.com/working-remote/#30f3de8e413f
https://www.forbes.com/forbeswomen/#29642e41621e

I realize this topic wasn't touched on much throughout the course of the book, but not because I didn't feel it deserves attention. There are so many considerations regarding children, parenting, homeschooling, activities, and more that the topic deserves its own book. These are just a small sample of some of the resources my friends who are parents have mentioned. You may also wish to network with other parents through LinkedIn, Facebook groups and blogs, as the community effort is strong.

And if you're hitting the road soon, take a look at these offerings:
Connectivity:
https://www.opensignal.com/
https://faroutride.com/internet-vanlife/
https://www.chasingthewildgoose.com/vanlife-wifi-options/
https://vanliving101.com/2019/09/30/create-your-own-secured-wifi-hotspot-in-your-van/

The first link is a helpful map that I found a little too late for my own benefit, which is why I share it here. Open Signal can help you figure out where you can get a cellphone and WiFi signal, based on your carrier. This is the type of information you should consult before you plan a day of wandering, especially if you have a deadline creeping up.

The other three links are expert Van Lifer accounts of different ways you can access WiFi on the road.

Please note: Technology changes every day. These links are contemporary to the publication of this book, and may or may not be helpful at the time of your specific voyage.

Putting an Office in Your Van:
https://www.parkedinparadise.com/mobile-office/
https://www.youtube.com/watch?v=5JEN5zcnc40

https://pursuitist.com/office-on-wheels-for-those-who-love-to-work-on-the-go/
https://www.technicallywizardry.com/mobile-office-desk-van/

Ultimately, how you fit your office into your van, skoolie, RV, or camper is going to depend on the space you have, your carpentry and creating skills, and your overall grand plan. I wanted to provide a few links to those who have done it, though, so you can gain inspiration and rest assured that it can be done.

Recommended Reading For Making It Work:
http://thevanual.com/working-and-living/
https://divineontheroad.com/van-life-remote-jobs/
https://www.outsideonline.com/2316796/i-gave-my-house-vanlife-while-holding-down-9-5
https://marcysutton.com/remote-work-van-life

It may seem strange that I'm including other people's blogs in my book, but #VanLife isn't just a lifestyle, it's a community. I wanted to take the opportunity to demonstrate that there are other people who do this, and to provide you with the chance to get their perspective on the matter. Again, I couldn't include links to every single Van Lifer's thoughts on the matter, but I encourage anyone considering this to read anything they can from people who have been there and done that. Don't just take my word for it!

Network/Community Resources

Maintaining community is a strong instinct within human nature, and one that we use to our advantage. We crave the support and interaction of sympathetic parties. These sites are designed to help motivate remote workers, and alleviate some of the growing pains by connecting you with others who are wandering down similar paths.

I'd also like to mention that LinkedIn, Facebook, and Reddit are all great community resources for multiple reasons. Forums are not without opinions of course, so join discussions at your own risk, but the "real people talking about real things" model is something that has helped many people feel comfortable with their challenges and not so alone.

I've tried to include a little something for everyone here, since we touched on many different scenarios in the course of the book.

For Women:
Power to Fly: https://powertofly.com/
Remote Woman: https://remotewoman.com/community/
TED for Women: https://www.ted.com/topics/women+in+business
Women Entrepreneur: https://www.entrepreneur.com/women
It pains me to say it, but even today, women are met with a different set of challenges in the workforce. These sites provide connections to jobs, to resources to support and guide, and access to a community of women who face similar situations.

For Side Hustlers:
Believe In A Budget: https://believeinabudget.com/
Side Hustle Nation: https://www.facebook.com/groups/sidehustlenation/
Side Hustle School: https://sidehustleschool.com/
All of these represent useful tools for getting started with your side hustle. I've included some blogs, some podcasts, some training tools, and idea generators. Again, not an exhaustive list, but certainly one that should get the brain focused on making this happen!

For Freelancers:
Freelance Lift: https://www.freelancelift.com/
Freelancers' Union: https://www.freelancersunion.org/
The Middle Finger Project Blog: https://www.themiddlefingerproject.org/blog/
One Woman Shop- A Solopreneur Community and Resource Hub: https://onewomanshop.com/
Again, there are thousands of resources for freelancers to join minds with other freelancers. I wanted to include a few blogs and communities to allow a variety of points of view on this topic. Each of these links leads to plenty of thoughts, opinions, experiences, and regular daily commentary

on the reality of freelancing, along with valuable resources for those of us living the dream.

For Corporate Workers:
Virtual Vocations: https://www.virtualvocations.com/blog/
The Remote Work Summit: https://www.theremoteworksummit.com/
Work Remotely: https://slofile.com/slack/workremotely
Remote Work Slack: https://remoteworkslack.com/?ref=workfrom.co/chat
While it may not be exactly the same as doing shots at the bar within walking distance of the office, these communities, blogs, and resources can help re-energize the social needs within you. Plus, you'll get the chance to banter, vent, bemoan, and learn without a hefty bar bill.

For Those Working from the Road:
Project Van Life Forum: https://forum.projectvanlife.com/
Vanlife Magazine Forum: https://vanlifemagazine.co/
The Vanlife App: https://www.thevanlifeapp.com/
Kristine Hudson's Facebook Group: https://www.facebook.com/eternalvantrip/
These are just a few of the online communities available for folks, including my own fledgling Facebook community. While these forums cover a variety of topics relevant to anyone who's home has wheels, work, productivity, and money are definitely amongst those topics. Plus, if you don't see what you need to know, start a thread!

If you know of a good link, resource, or helpful community, feel free to share it on my official Facebook page. After all, you're never alone!

Reviews

Reviews and feedback help improve this book and the author. If you enjoy this book, we would greatly appreciate it if you could take a few moments to share your opinion and post a review on Amazon.

www.ingramcontent.com/pod-product-compliance
Lightning Source LLC
Chambersburg PA
CBHW051542020426
42333CB00016B/2055